T0134055

Creating Life from Life

Creating Life from Life

Biotechnology and Science Fiction

edited by
Rosalyn W. Berne

PAN STANFORD PUBLISHING

Published by

Pan Stanford Publishing Pte. Ltd.
Penthouse Level, Suntec Tower 3
8 Temasek Boulevard
Singapore 038988

Email: editorial@panstanford.com
Web: www.panstanford.com

British Library Cataloguing-in-Publication Data
A catalogue record for this book is available from the British Library.

Creating Life from Life: Biotechnology and Science Fiction

ISBN 978-981-4463-58-4 (Hardcover)
ISBN 978-981-4463-59-1 (eBook)

Printed in the USA

To

Dr. Roland A. and *Mrs. Muriel D. Wiggins*

Contents

About the Editor

Dr. Rosalyn W. Berne is an associate professor of science, technology, and society in the Department of Engineering & Society at the University of Virginia. She explores the intersecting realms between emerging technologies, science, fiction, and myth and between the human and nonhuman worlds, and the ethical implications of technological development. Of particular interest to her are the roles and functions of moral imagination, personal belief, mythology, and metaphor in the pursuit of technological development. Seeing the capacity of science fiction to provoke reflection and moral imagination, she both writes and teaches in that genre. Dr. Berne is the author of *When the Horses Whisper* (Rainbow Ridge Books, 2013), a nonfiction treatise on animal communication; *Waiting in the Silence* (Spore Press, 2012), a science fiction novel (nominated for the Virginia Library Annual Literary Award); and *Nanotalk: Conversations with Scientists and Engineers about Ethics, Meaning and Belief in the Development of Nanotechnology* (Erlbaum, 2005). She has authored six of the companion short stories included in this book.

Acknowledgments

Many thanks go to the scientists, historians, philosophers of science, and students who contributed essays to this collection. Obviously, the book would not have been possible without their participation. To my husband, William Prindle, I offer my heartfelt appreciation for his most helpful, often late-night readings of the short stories and the keen suggestions he made, and to Kathleen Manuel, who as usual offered timely and astute editing support. The Science, Technology, and Society program in the School of Engineering and Applied Sciences of the University of Virginia, as my academic home, continues to nurture my intellectual curiosities. My deepest appreciation goes to Bernard Carlson, chair of the Department of Engineering and Society, who supported this project, in particular, and the writing retreat I needed to complete it. Deborah Johnson, immediate past chair of the department, and my colleagues there continue to offer their fine fellowship. I thank you all wholeheartedly.

Chapter 1

Introduction: Dialectic of Scientific Writing and Science Fiction

Rosalyn W. Berne

Technology and Society Department of Engineering and Society School of Engineering and Applied Science, PO Box 400744, University of Virginia, Charlottesville, VA 22904, USA

rwb@virginia.edu

Much hope rests in the pursuit of biotechnology.

There are more than 300 million people in the world living with diabetes. Though treatable when diagnosed, diabetes has long-term complications, such as increased risk for cardiovascular disease. Diabetes has been reversed in mice through human stem cell implants (Palmer, 2012).

Both the elderly and children can experience macular degeneration leading to significant vision loss. The cure for blindness may have been science fiction, when the sight-restoring visor worn by *Star Trek*'s character Geordi La Forge was replaced by ocular prosthetic implants. But gene therapy, stem cell therapy, and a genetically modified version of vitamin A are currently being researched as viable cures. And scientists have grown the precursor of the human eye in the laboratory (Cyranoski, 2012).

Creating Life from Life: Biotechnology and Science Fiction
Edited by Rosalyn W. Berne
Copyright © 2015 Pan Stanford Publishing Pte. Ltd.
ISBN 978-981-4463-58-4 (Hardcover), 978-981-4463-59-1 (eBook)
www.panstanford.com

Many, many millions of people around the world are addicted to nicotine. Nicotine is extremely addictive. The addiction is, in large measure, why cigarette use is so common from young teen smokers to the elderly. But the habit is known to be deadly. In the United States alone, cigarette smoking results in more than 443,000 premature deaths a year. We may be approaching the time when a simple vaccine will treat nicotine addiction. Scientists are experimenting with the use of mice liver for the production of antibodies that consume nicotine the moment it enters the bloodstream, before it ever has a chance to reach the brain or the heart (Weil Medical College, 2012).

Biotechnology involves the manipulation of biological macromolecules or organisms in experimental procedures in order to create useful products and applications in the agricultural, pharmaceutical, health, and allied industries. The potential cures for diabetes, blindness, and nicotine addiction are given above as examples of medical biotechnology. Gene therapy, drug production, and genetic testing all are outgrowths of biotechnology. Closely aligned to biotechnology is bioengineering, which involves the interface of technology with living systems, for similar purposes. In agriculture, biotechnology is applied for crop yield increases, reduced vulnerability to drought, and enhancement of nutritional properties of plants.

The terms "bionanotechnology," "nanobiotechnology," and "nanobiology" all refer to the intersection of nanotechnology with biology, nanotechnology being a science that takes place at the scale of a billionth of a meter. The convergence of biotechnology with nanotechnology, information, and cognitive sciences is referred to as NBIC.

The outgrowth of these burgeoning fields of biotechnology research represents a far-reaching range of potential applications limited, perhaps, only by human imagination: From exogenesis (the gestation of pregnancy outside the womb) to sex selection; from pharmacogenomics (the adaption of drugs to the particular genome of an individual) to biological weapons; and from human bone made from skins cells to cord blood cells for treatment of neurological diseases, biotechnology is fueling our current technological revolution.

The biotechnology revolution was launched on a global scale many decades ago and, through the manipulation and control of biological processes, has taken a direct course toward creating life. Yet there are still many choices to be made in shaping the futures that may be made possible through biotechnology. Where this research is leading, and what this revolution will mean to human society, to the earth's ecosystems, and to other living species, has not yet been determined. Market demands, regulatory processes, ethical queries, narratives, and storytelling all will play a role in how we construe what it means to be autonomous agents in interaction with one another, as biotechnology makes its way deep into the fabric of our lives. What, for example, would it mean if before their birth, we could select which physical and emotional characteristics we'd like our children to have and then once they are born could decide whether to enhance their mental capacities either biochemically or with biomedical devices embedded in their brains? That may sound like science fiction but perhaps so only for the time being.

The word "revolution" is often used in reference to the emergence of dramatic new technological capabilities. Whether one creates these new capabilities, or simply benefits from their use, or even feels victimized by them (such as the Luddites of 19th-century England), the meaning of the word resonates with significance. Like the Cultural Revolution of 1960s' China, and the counterculture revolution of the 1960s' United States, the word "revolution" generally suggests the overthrow or repudiation of an established order or system. Any radical or pervasive change in society may be labeled a revolution. So it's no surprise that major technological shifts would also be seen in this way, since by its nature technology changes society, even as society gives rise to it.

With the Neolithic Revolution came the introduction of agriculture, the domestication of animals, and a more sedentary human life cycle. These changes heralded a shift away from humans' original hunting and gathering cultures. In a similar way, the Industrial Revolution in Europe, with its unprecedented and rapid promulgation of technology, launched a shift from human and animal labor to the work of machines. The introduction of the steam engine and the rise of manufacturing transformed the world in unpredicted and radical ways. The information revolution, which continues to unfold today, has created still more astonishing shifts in economic, technological, and social systems. Our major systems of commerce, education, health care, government, and warfare depend almost entirely on electronic forms of information. Biotechnology also has revolutionary implications, too, in that its effects may be unknowable, reaching well beyond any we might predict.

We stand today on the brink of yet another technological revolution, this one occurring at the intersections of nano-, bio-, and information technologies with cognitive sciences, radical changes loom. If this impending technological revolution is seen in terms of warfare, like a line of soldiers moving rapidly in our direction, but beyond our control, then the word "revolution" is apt. In this case it implies that inexorable forces will produce gains for some and losses for others. If, on the other hand, we choose to see the coming changes in terms of intentional and conscious design, then perhaps the term "technological creation" might better connote the possibilities of what we humans intend to create in this next phase.

Dialectic as a Discourse of Change

The practice of biotechnology is a scientific endeavor but is also a social one. As we continue to pursue scientific and technological knowledge and capabilities, many scholars, scientists, and citizens around the world are engaged in an inquiry on how we, as individuals and as society, might best guide our choices. While "pure" research is said to be pursued as knowledge for its own sake, technologies are created for very particular purposes, often to address societal problems, alleviate human suffering, or seek militaristic and economic gains. Now, at the brink of rapidly emerging, potent biotechnological capabilities, it is essential that we intelligently and conscientiously question our purposes and intentions, attentive to the well-being of humanity, our fellow creatures, and the earth.*

Borrowing from the language of linguist Norman Fairclough, biotechnology involves instruments, objects, practices, values, forms of consciousness, and discourses and is interconnected to family life, economics, religion, culture, and politics. All these are dialectically related, meaning that although they appear to exist discreetly, they do not function as "objects versus subjects" (i.e., science vs. science fiction). Rather, they are connected as a medium by which truth may be revealed in our striving to define reality. Given the transformative nature of the biotechnology revolution, our reality will need to be continually redefined.

In laying out a dialectic theory of discourse, Fairclough (2001) argues that language has qualitatively different significance in contemporary socioeconomic changes than in previous transformations. This is because on the basis of important new technologies, language has become knowledge based and knowledge driven. He further suggests that "the relationship between discourse and other elements of social practices is a dialectical relationship," (Fairclough, 2001, p. 3) which I think would be especially true for the social practice that biotechnology is. As an evocative form of discourse used in many cultures, science fiction has functioned to help us define our changing reality. Even as far back as 1817, Mary Shelly's *Frankenstein* was published at the brink of the Industrial Revolution, when Galvanism and the seemingly incredible power of electricity

---

*As was suggested by philosopher Jacques Ellul's "76 Reasonable Questions to Ask about Any Technology." (See the appendix for the complete list.)

spurred the imagination. Today the story continues to have mythological significance as the biotechnological revolution gains momentum. In Fairclough's terminology, biotechnology "internalizes and is internalized by" science fictional forms of discourse without "being reducible to each other." He writes:

> Of course knowledge (science, technology) have long been significant factors in economic and social change, but what is being pointed to is a dramatic increase in their significance. The relevance of these ideas here is that knowledge-driven amounts to discourse-driven: knowledges are generated and circulate as discourses, and the process through which discourses become operationalized in economies and societies is precisely the dialectics of discourse. (p. 3)

And since, as Fairclough explains, those dialectics of discourse "include representations of how things are and have been, as well as imaginaries in representations of how things might or could or should be," both biotechnology and science fiction function as projections of possible states of being inside of possible new worlds.

Mar and Oatley (2008) draw a parallel between fiction and simulation claiming, "The abstraction performed by fictional stories demands that readers and others project themselves into the represented events. The function of fiction can thus be seen to include the recording, abstraction, and communication of complex social information in a manner that offers personal enactments of experience, rendering it more comprehensible than usual" (p. 173).

Following Nelson Goodman's general thesis that "symbolic systems make and remake the world" and Mary Hesse's interpretation of scientific models as "sustained metaphors aiming at re-description of reality," philosopher Paul Riceour places fiction inside a theory of imagination as "reality shaping." Fiction changes reality by both inventing and discovering it. Riceour (1979) writes:

> The ultimate role of the image is not only to diffuse meaning across diverse sensorial fields, to hallucinate thought in some way, but on the contrary to effect a sort of Epoché of the real, to suspend our attention to the real, to place us in a state of non-engagement with regard to perception or action, in short, to suspend meaning in the neutralized atmosphere to which one could give the name of the dimension of fiction. In this state of non-engagement we try new ideas, new values, new ways of being-in-the-world. Imagination is this free play of possibilities. In this state, fiction can, as we said above, create a re-description of reality. (p. 134)

As such, science fiction and biotechnology make for compelling companions in a dialectic that considers the creation of our world. The imaginative work of science fiction can serve to both predict and experiment with possible futures of our sociobiotechnical existence, extrapolating from the present into worlds yet to come, to be experienced directly by the reader.

Science fiction author David Brin (2008) writes, "Many people have tried to define science fiction. I like to call it the literature of exploration and change. While other genres obsess upon so-called eternal verities, science fiction deals with the possibility that our children may have different problems. They may, indeed, be different than we have been" (p. 186). Biotechnology, also imaginative, explores, alters, and experiments with life forms for use in creating applications that can enhance and improve the quality of human life.

This capacity to manipulate and create new life reflects the expansiveness of human knowledge and ambition. As our curiosity deepens, our imagination magnifies, and our scientific tools become increasingly sophisticated, we more readily are able and inclined to move into the cells, the molecules, and even onto the DNA itself, manipulating these to create life from life.

By eliciting moral imagination, science fiction, when paired with scientific writing, can provide a means not only of making predictions but also of creatively considering core questions regarding the implications of science and technology: What is it we value? What is it we mean to be? What may we be able to do? What do we want to accomplish? How will technology help or hinder us in providing meaningful answers to these questions? If we fail to temper the biotechnological revolution with moral imagination, we may find ourselves caught in an increasingly unrecognizable world where our choices shrink beyond our grasp. Through its capacity to bring forth an awareness of its social implications, science fiction can be an important beacon for guiding the incredibly creative endeavors of biotechnology. In dialectic with scientific writing, we open to more conscientious, creative pursuits.

Overview of Contributors

Creating Life from Life: Biotechnology and Science Fiction features a collection of essays written by scientists who are engaged in biotechnology research, explaining and expressing some of their interests, curiosities, and concerns. Science fiction short stories serve as companion pieces to the scientists' essays. The intention is to spawn dialectic, sparking the moral imagination of the reader in contemplation of what we may one day be and what it may mean to be human as our biotechnological endeavors continue to evolve. On the belief science is contributing profoundly to the continual creation our own destiny, my hope is that the combination of these essays and stories will be synergistic in the process of determining who it is we intend to become, and what it is we aim to create, through the tools of the biotechnology revolution.

The book begins with a history of biotechnology, written by Dr. Catherine Rhodes. Dr. Rhodes is a research fellow in science ethics for the Institute for Science, Ethics and Innovation at the University of Manchester, specializing in the international regulations relevant to control of biotechnology. Her research is motivated by the concern that while science has the potential to make substantial contributions to addressing the major challenges faced by humanity, it is currently impeded from doing so by a range of factors and dynamics operating internationally. Dr. Rhodes has a particular interest in the governance of genetic resources and associated data, which has important implications for the use of biological sciences in managing challenges such as food security, climate change adaptation and mitigation, and responses to emerging disease threats. Her "History of the Biotechnology Revolution" is placed as the book's opening essay to provide the reader with a thorough background of biotechnology development. What follows are essays by individual scientists working in fields related to biotechnology, each with companion science fiction stories to place the essays into an imaginative perspective of human life.

Dr. Eduardo A. Nillni writes on the subject of obesity. Obesity and its related medical complications, including type 2 diabetes, cardiovascular disease, dyslipidemia, and cancer, account for more than 300,000 deaths per year in the United States. Obesity occurs as a result of a long-standing imbalance between energy intake and energy expenditure, which is influenced by a very complex set of biological pathway systems regulating appetite. Dr. Nillni's laboratory studies the biology of different hypothalamic neuropeptide hormones and enzyme nutrient sensors involved in the regulation of energy balance. Dr. Nillni is a member of the research faculty in the Division of Endocrinology in the Department of Medicine at Brown University. He is also an appointed member of the Integrative Physiology of Obesity and Diabetes National Institutes of Health Study Section (IPOD). He was the recipient of the 2001 Bruce Selya Award for Research Excellence at Lifespan, and his work was featured in a National Science Foundation progress report to the US Congress. His contribution, "The Cycle of Obesity," is followed by the companion science fiction short story "Madeline."

Dr. Joel A. Pedersen is a professor in the Department of Soil Science at the University of Madison, Wisconsin. Dr. Pedersen's research group studies physicochemical and biophysical processes affecting the behavior of organic molecules, biomolecules, and nanoparticles in terrestrial and aquatic environments, emphasizing quantitative and mechanistic studies of the interaction of organic contaminants and macromolecules with environmental interfaces. One of his research topics is the environmental transmission of prion diseases, a family of brain-wasting diseases that infect humans and other mammals. "Prion Diseases," his contribution to this volume, explains the disease's symptoms, the processes governing the environmental transmission of the disease's existence in nonhuman animals, its transmission to other hosts, and the potential for it to reach humans. Following Pedersen's essay is a companion science fiction short story entitled "Carnivore's Game."

Dr. David L. Feldman is a professor and chair of the Department of Planning, Policy, and Design and adjunct professor of political science in the School of Ecology at the University of California Irvine. He specializes in water resources management and policy, global climate change policy, ethics and environmental decisions, adaptive management, and sustainable development. His current research is focused on the sources of value conflicts over allocation and distribution of water and the difficulties in achieving institutional reform to promote equity in water management in the United States and elsewhere. In his contributing chapter, "Climate Change and the Future of Freshwater," Dr. Feldman posits a not-too-distant future where rain and snow patterns have shifted as a result of human activities. His essay offers a reflection on global climate change and water-related extreme climate events that will require our adaptation. Dr. Feldman offers hope in the fact that such adaptations are already occurring; local communities, NGOs, scientists, and aid organizations are working together to design solutions, identify funding sources, and share vital information. Dr. Feldman's essay is followed by the companion science fiction short story "Negotiations."

Dr. Shayn Peirce-Cottler is an associate professor of biomedical engineering at the University of Virginia, and she has a joint appointment in the Department of Ophthalmology. She researches the microvasculature—a complex network of highly specialized blood vessels, capable of growing and altering its structure and function to regulate blood flow and accommodate the changing metabolic needs of the body's tissues. Microvascular growth and remodeling are important in pathological conditions, such as wound healing, ischemic disease (e.g., peripheral vascular disease and heart disease), and tumor growth. She studies microvascular growth and remodeling using novel computational and experimental techniques, including agent-based computational models and thin tissues that enable visualization and manipulation of entire microvascular networks in vivo. Her research group also develops therapeutic approaches to grow and regenerate injured and diseased tissues by manipulating the structure and composition of the microvasculature using cell therapies and novel drugs. Her essay, "Stems Cells to Cure Diabetes-Induced Vision Loss," explains the findings of one such project. "Shadows and Sugars and Shades of Gray (Madeline, Part 2)" follows as its companion science fiction short story.

Reginald H. Garrett is a professor of biology at the University of Virginia. Dr. Garrett's areas of research include biochemistry, molecular biology, and metabolism. He and his colleague Mitchell Smith of the Center for Food Safety and Applied Nutrition (CFSAN) in the Food and Drug Administration (FDA) are seeking to discover the relationship between inflammatory disease conditions and the consumption of various drugs and/ or dietary supplements, such as eosinophilia-myalgia syndrome (EMS) and the consumption of L-tryptophan-containing dietary supplements (LTCDS). Dr. Garrett has contributed two essays. The first, "Neogenesis," recounts the creation of self-replicating synthetic bacterial cells and provides a brief overview of how DNA works. He explains how it is possible to type out the genetic code for a new organism, synthesize it chemically, and express it in an appropriate cell cytoplasm, leading to neogenesis, the creation of new life. The essay ends with the rhetorical question, how will governments and industries ever discover a stolen secret encoded as DNA? That question is explored in a companion science fiction short story entitled "Madness Enough to Break the World," written by Dr. Sean Hays. Dr. Garrett's second essay contribution, "Who Do They Think They Are?," pits social assumptions about the validity of race against the scientific implausibility of race as a human characteristic of significant distinction. "Emmanuel," an excerpt from the book *Waiting in the Silence*, is offered as its science fiction companion piece.

Dr. Hays is currently a *postdoktor* at the University of Bergen in Norway, where he is studying posthuman warfare, lethal autonomous robots, and the emergent properties of new military and intelligence strategy and weapons systems. He was formerly a postdoctoral fellow with the Consortium for Science, Policy, and Outcomes at its DC location and a postdoctoral fellow at the Center for Nanotechnology in Society at Arizona State University. As a Future Tense researcher at the New America Foundation, Dr. Hays has worked to design and coordinate the Future Tense initiative, an attempt at public and policymaker engagement on the governance of emergent technology. His research has focused on the impact of emergent technologies on social competition in US political culture. His dissertation is a preliminary analysis of the implications of cognitive enhancement technologies in that same context. He is the lead editor of *Nanotechnology, the Brain and the Future* (Springer, 2013) and of a book about creating a system for modeling nonlinear dynamic technological histories. Dr. Hays helped design, field, and analyze the first nationally representative survey on nanotechnology and neuroscience. He is a novelist, writing in the genres of science fiction and cyberpunk.

Dr. Elizabeth Hood has more than 35 years of experience in biology. She is currently a distinguished professor of agriculture at Arkansas State University (ASU). With three partners, she has started a company to produce enzymes for biomass conversion from transgenic plants. She runs an active research lab at ASU in plant-based protein production technology and cell wall structure and function. Dr. Hood was a program director in molecular and cellular biosciences at the National Science Foundation during 2003–2004. She was a leader in forming one of the world's foremost transgenic plant research groups at ProdiGene, a plant biotechnology company. Dr. Hood is internationally recognized for her research program and associated expertise, as evidenced by over 90 publications and patents, as well as invitations to speak nationally and internationally. Her research interests are in the areas of renewable resources, foreign gene expression in transgenic plants, plant cell wall structure and function, and protein targeting. She has expertise in deconstructing plant cell walls with custom cocktails of enzymes produced in her own plant-based production system. Dr. Hood has contributed the essay "Keys to Bioproducts from Agriculture." The short story "Soon They Will Know Our Secrets" follows.

Dr. David Carmel is a cognitive neuroscientist. He holds degrees in medical science, psychology, and interdisciplinary humanities and a PhD in psychology from University College London. He is currently a lecturer in psychology at the University of Edinburgh. His main research interests are consciousness, how the brain creates it, and how it interacts with faculties such as attention and memory. His lab employs various techniques to address these questions, including magnetic brain stimulation and neuroimaging. His ideas on the brain and mind have appeared in *Scientific American Mind* and fivebooks.com. Dr. Carmel has contributed the essay "The Promise and Pitfalls of Cognitive Enhancement" and his own companion science fiction short story, "Dr. Hyde."

Dr. Nathaniel Cady's research group at the State University of New York, Albany, focuses on the unique interface between nanotechnology and biology. Nanotechnology is engineering scaled at approximately one-billionth of a meter, and Dr. Cady's interest is in how nanoscale devices, materials, or phenomena can be harnessed for therapeutics, diagnostics, medicine, pharmaceuticals, and other biological applications. Drawing knowledge from biological systems enables unique approaches to such capacities. "Build Me a Memory," his own science fiction tale, tells a story about neuromorphic computing, which closely mimics the processes of the human brain. In the world he extrapolates from current research, brain–computer interfaces have made possible computers that not only think like us but also are part of us.

Dr. Catherine Rhodes's second contribution, "The Uncertain Consequences of the Biotechnology Revolution," provides a sense of what may be at stake as "the revolution" continues to unfold. "Rōnin," a short story written by Lena Nguyen, propels the questions of social-ethical consequences of the biotechnology revolution, out to the far reaches of human-created, human-like life.

A graduate of Barrett, the Honors College at Arizona State University, Nguyen pursued a double major in English (creative writing) as well as political science and international relations. She is now enrolled in an MFA program for Creative Writing at Cornell University. Born in 1992, she is the daughter of Vietnamese immigrants, and from an early age, she discovered her love of English, writing, literature, and fiction. She began her college career at the age of 12, studying at the University of California, Los Angeles (UCLA), Stanford University, Brown University, and Harvard University, and pursued a wide range of academic fields: behavioral psychology, astronomy, political science, and, above all, the art of writing fiction. She has won numerous writing competitions and published her first short story in *The Harvard Review*. Nguyen's dream is to become a science fiction and fantasy novelist.

References

Brin, D. (2003). Tomorrow may be different, in *Exploring the Matrix: Visions of the Cyber Present*. Haber, K. (ed.), 186. New York, NY: Macmillan.

Weil Medical College (June 27, 2012). New vaccine for nicotine addiction. Weill Cornell researchers develop novel anti-body vaccine that blocks addictive nicotine chemicals from reaching the brain. Press release. Cornell, NY: Weil Medical College.

Cyranoski, D. (2012). Biologists grow human-eye precursor from stem cells. *Nature,* http://www.nature.com/news/biologists-grow-human-eye-precursor-from-stem-cells-1.10835.

Fairclough, N. (2001). The dialectics of discourse. *Textus*, **14**(2), 3–10, http://www.sfu.ca/cmns/courses/2012/801/1-Readings/Fairclough%20 Dialectics%20of%20Discourse%20Analysis.pdf.

Mar, R. A., and Oatley, K. (2008). The function of fiction is the abstraction and simulation of social experience. *Perspectives on Psychological Science*, 3(3), 173–192. doi:10.1111/j.1745-6924.2008.00073.x.

Palmer, R. (2012). Diabetes reversed in mice thanks to stem cell transplant. *International Business Times*, http://www.ibtimes.com/diabetes-reversed-mice-thanks-stem-cell-transplant-704558.

Riceour, P. (1979). The function of fiction in shaping reality, *Man and World*, **11–12**, 1978–1979.

Tolman, C. (1983). Further comments on the meaning of "dialectic." *Human Development*, **26**, 320–324.

Chapter 2

History of the Biotechnology Revolution

Catherine Rhodes

Institute for Science, Ethics and Innovation, Faculty of Life Sciences,
University of Manchester, Oxford Road, Manchester,
M13 9PL, UK
catherine.rhodes-2@manchester.ac.uk

The biotechnology revolution is based on massive scientific advances that have been made over the last 60 years. These advances have given scientists an extremely detailed understanding of life processes, have allowed life forms to be deliberately manipulated at the genetic level, and have enabled the creation of novel organisms containing genes from other species. To understand the history of the biotechnology revolution, it is useful to look at the development of the science that has helped to create it. There was a significant merging of chemistry and biology (still seen by many as two distinct strands of science) in the early 1950s as connections were made between the molecular structure of deoxyribonucleic acid (DNA) and its role in inheritance. The revolutionary techniques of genetic engineering and genome sequencing stem from this convergence.

Creating Life from Life: Biotechnology and Science Fiction
Edited by Rosalyn W. Berne
Copyright © 2015 Pan Stanford Publishing Pte. Ltd.
ISBN 978-981-4463-58-4 (Hardcover), 978-981-4463-59-1 (eBook)
www.panstanford.com

This chapter recounts the history of chemistry and the history of genetics separately until 1953 (but this is not to suggest that there was no earlier interaction between the two), before looking at the development of genetic engineering and genome sequencing from then until the present day. The scientific advances have rapidly and often quite directly found applications in a variety of products and processes since the mid-1970s. This chapter, therefore, also looks briefly at the history of biotechnology applications.

Chemistry in 1770–1953

The links between the development of modern chemistry and modern biotechnology may not be immediately apparent. However, new discoveries and techniques in chemistry have been vitally important to the development of modern biotechnology, and the two areas continue to be connected. Of greatest importance was the discovery of the molecular structure (and from this the chemical properties) of deoxyribonucleic acid (DNA). James Watson and Francis Crick discovered the structure of DNA in 1953. At this point the fields of chemistry and biology merged in significant ways to produce the tools, techniques, and knowledge that drive the biotechnology revolution. A lot of important steps had to be taken in the field of chemistry before scientists were able to define complex molecular structures like DNA, and these will be looked at briefly in this section.

Modern chemistry is usually dated as emerging in the 1770s with the discrediting of the established phlogiston theory.* One scientist, in particular, is considered to have been instrumental in this move to modern chemistry—Lavoisier, who, using the newly refined concept of elements, came up with the chemical atomic theory that "different elements have fundamentally different atoms" (Hudson, 1992, p. 77). He and others then worked on

---

*A chemical theory of the eighteenth century, which postulated that flammable materials released a substance known as phlogiston when burned.

identifying as many of these elements as possible. Lavoisier listed 31 elements in his 1789 book *Elements of Chemistry* (another chemist, Berzelius, listed 49 in 1826). However, chemical atomic theory was not widely taken up or much used until the periodic table was established—Mendeleev first published his periodic table in 1869—and this was not to be achieved until there had been some agreement between chemists on atomic and molecular weights. An international congress of chemists was called in 1860, seeking to clarify issues on the establishment of atomic and molecular weights. Although no agreement was reached at the congress it did provide the impetus for the resolution of these issues, which occurred during the following decade.

The study of chemistry split between organic and inorganic chemistry around 1860. Organic chemistry concerns compounds containing carbon, whereas inorganic chemistry concerns those that do not. This was a split more in the focus of research than in techniques, and the two areas remain connected. The establishment of atomic weights brought progress to both areas, allowing the periodic table to be formed and also enabling molecular formulae to be deduced. The formulae of molecules are important in identifying their structure. Knowledge of the atomic weights of elements allowed their proportions within molecules to be worked out.

The discovery of further elements continued well into the twentieth century. Mendeleev had left gaps in his periodic table at points where he had predicted these elements would fall. Two techniques aided the discovery of new elements. The first, developed in 1860, used a spectroscope that could be used to analyze light produced from burning materials (Hudson, 1992, p. 125). Several elements were discovered in this way that had previously been hard to identify due to their being present only in tiny amounts mixed up with other materials. The second and better-known technique was developed in 1898 by Marie and Pierre Curie, who made use of radioactivity to discover new elements, including radium and polonium, through their radioactive isotopes. Increasing knowledge of relatively simple molecular structures enabled increased work to take place on the synthesis of organic compounds from inorganic elements. This had first been shown to be possible in 1828 with the synthesis of urea, but knowledge of molecular structure enabled it to take place more systematically. Soon chemists were also "producing compounds that had no natural counterparts" (Hudson, 1992, p. 144), particularly dyes and drugs.

As more was discovered about the structure of simple molecules, chemists were able to progress to working out the more complicated structures of some of the larger, complex molecules that existed in nature. It was work in this area that was to lead to the discovery of the structure of DNA.

A new technique of X-ray crystallography, developed in 1913, was to enable the identification of the structures of much larger molecules. This technique essentially allowed a photograph of a molecule to be produced from its crystalline form, by making use of X-ray diffraction, that is, the way X-rays are deflected from their original course when they hit the molecule. This technique was refined over the following decades, allowing sharper images to be produced. Such a picture of DNA, produced by Rosalind Franklin in 1952, gave Watson and Crick significant clues about its structure. There was also an obstacle of how to deal with the large amounts of information that would be produced when dealing with more complex molecules containing thousands of atoms. The invention of electronic computers helped to overcome this obstacle (Hudson, 1992, p. 224).

Other discoveries about the chemistry of DNA had also assisted Watson and Crick, particularly the discovery by Erwin Chargraff that the number of adenine (A) bases was equal to the number of thymine (T) bases and the number of guanine (G) bases was equal to the number of cytosine (C) bases. Franklin also suggested (on the basis of her photograph) that the sugar–phosphate "backbone" of DNA ran along its outside. Further discoveries about the chemical properties of DNA and how it functions followed. Those are dealt with later in this chapter.

Developments in modern chemistry from the late eighteenth century onward enabled the structure of DNA to be worked out in 1953. Knowledge of the structure, properties, and functions of DNA, combined with the realization in the field of genetics that DNA carried heredity information, allowed new techniques of genetic engineering to be rapidly developed, and these techniques underpin the biotechnology revolution.

Genetics in 1900–1953

Many of the modern developments in biotechnology are based on a detailed knowledge of genes and genetics. This knowledge has been built up over the past century. Modern genetics study is said to have begun in 1900 with the rediscovery of Mendel's work on the inheritance of factors in pea plants (factors later to be termed "genes"). Mendel had published his work in 1866, but it attracted little attention until three scientists independently discovered the same principles (Carl Correns, Hugo de Vries, and Erich Von Tschermark) in 1900. Study of cells (cytology), aided by improvements in the clarity and magnification of microscopes, had led to the observation of chromosomes in 1879, and by 1900 it had also been shown that proteins and nucleic acids were present within cells. Through experimentation in the early twentieth century it was established that genes were located on the chromosomes. However, it was not until 1952 that it was widely accepted amongst geneticists that DNA carried genetic information; the proteins in cells had seemed better candidates for this role.

Acceptance of the role of DNA combined with the new knowledge of its molecular structure (announced by Watson and Crick in 1953) was to bring about the rapid development of new tools and techniques in genetic engineering, which in turn brought huge advances in biotechnology. Following Darwin's work on evolution (*Origin of the Species* was published in 1859) many people sought to discover how characteristics could be passed on from parents to offspring. These were suggested to be "material factors" and were recognized by Hugo de Vries (writing in 1910) to be "the units which the science of heredity has to investigate. Just as physics and chemistry go back to molecules and atoms, the biological sciences have to penetrate these units in order to explain, by means of their combinations, the phenomena of the living world" (Fruton, 1972, p. 225). (The units in fact turned out to be molecules of DNA.)

By the end of the nineteenth century cytologists studying the behavior of chromosomes had observed the processes of mitosis and meiosis, different types of cell division, providing good evidence that these parts of the cell could carry genetic information. There was a mechanism for duplication, which occurred during routine cell division (mitosis), and there was also a mechanism that allowed for the inheritance of both parents' genes through a reduction in the number of chromosomes by half in meiosis (cell division in the germ cells), which then combined with the other parent's half set during reproduction.

Studies of genetic changes (mutations) in the early twentieth century provided further evidence about the role and functions of chromosomes and also of the location of genes upon them. Significant work was done with the fruit fly *Drosophila melanogaster*. This fly breeds quickly, and that meant that mutations could be studied through many generations. Experiments with mutations reinforced Mendel's theory that some characteristics were inherited separately from one another, but also showed that some were linked in inheritance. Thomas Hunt Morgan also observed (and named) the phenomenon of "crossing over." This is where sections of a pair of chromosomes swap with each other during meiosis, causing mutations to occur. Morgan realized that this might allow the locations of genes to be established, and A. H. Sturtevant used statistical study of mutations and the frequency of crossing-over to establish the relative positions of six genes on one of *Drosophila*'s chromosomes in 1913. He then produced the first chromosome or linkage map based on this. By 1925 Morgan's team had located 100 genes on *Drosophila*'s 4 chromosomes.

Mutations are very significant to the study of genetics, and methods were later developed to increase mutation rates through radiation and chemical means. The early work on chromosome mapping helped to lay the basis for later, more complex mapping of the genomes, including the Human Genome Project (HGP).

By the 1920s the concept of the gene as the unit of heredity had been established, the study of genetics was well underway, and it was understood that gene expression and inheritance relied on processes occurring within the chromosomes. There had also been some suggestion that mutations might occur due to interference in the production of enzymes.

Puzzles remained of how the cell used genetic information, where genetic instructions came from, and why the information was expressed differently in different cells despite the same chromosomes being present. The theory was that proteins were responsible. Proteins are present in the cell, and enzymes (which are a form of protein) are used in many cytological processes. There had been a suggestion as early as 1884 by the scientist Oskar Hartwig that "nuclein is the substance that is responsible . . . for the transmission of hereditary characteristics" (Aldridge, 1996, p. 7). But this view was largely ignored until the early 1950s, partly because of a theory called the "tetranucleotide hypothesis" put forward by Phoebus Levene in the 1930s.

This held that the four nucleotides of DNA (adenine, thymine, guanine, and cytosine) made up a string of repetitive code and were therefore incapable of carrying the complex code that would be needed for holding genetic instructions. Proteins did not have this problem. Proteins are a type of complex molecule known because of its structure as a "polypeptide chain." They are made up of amino acids, and "there are 20 amino acids commonly found in proteins" (Aldridge, 1996, p. 13), allowing the variation necessary to hold a long and complicated code.

It was also decided in the 1920s that genes (and therefore what they were made of) had to be autocatalytic, that is, able to make themselves replicate.

Geneticists tried, but failed, to come up with a satisfactory theory as to how proteins achieved this. Once the molecular structure of DNA was established its autocatalytic properties were self-evident as Watson and Crick noted: "It has not escaped our notice that the specific pairing we have postulated immediately suggests a possible copying mechanism for the genetic material" (Hudson, 1992, p. 225).

Further evidence of mutations being linked to a lack of a particular enzyme led to another theory (by Beadle and Tatum) that also hindered the recognition of the significance of DNA. The "one gene, one enzyme" hypothesis, while not essentially wrong, did lead some to the erroneous conclusion that enzymes were genes. The theory has since been revised to the "one gene, one polypeptide" hypothesis, but it was along the right lines— genes do code for enzymes. It was not until Chargraff did disprove the tetranucleotide hypothesis in 1948 that the possibility of DNA carrying genetic information was taken seriously. He showed through paper chromatography that the nucleotides did not form a repetitive sequence, and so it was possible for DNA to be carrying a code. Experiments on pneumococci bacteria by Oswald Avery in 1944 had shown that DNA was likely to be the "transforming principle" exchanged between bacteria and led to the statement that "nucleic acids of this type must be regarded not merely as structurally important but as functionally active in determining the biochemical activities and specific characteristics of pneumococcal cells" (Fruton, 1972, p. 248, quoting Avery, McLeod, and McCarty in 1944). Yet it seems to have been experiments on bacteriophages by Hershey and Chase (who published their findings in 1952) that finally convinced geneticists that DNA was the molecule of heredity. Using radioactive tags (one that attached only to DNA and one that attached only to protein) they showed that it was through the transference of

DNA that bacteriophages attack bacteria. Cytology combined with genetics to lead in just over half a century to the crucial discovery of the role of DNA in inheritance and its importance in the functioning of cells. Coupled with new knowledge about the molecular structure of DNA, this led to rapid development of new genetic engineering tools and techniques, which underpin the biotechnology revolution.

Genetic Engineering from 1953 Onward

By 1953 there was widespread acceptance among geneticists that DNA carried genetic information and its molecular structure had been discovered. This opened up the possibility that genes could be manipulated at the molecular level and their function understood and possibly corrected or controlled. First scientists had to work out how genes are expressed, that is, how DNA codes for proteins. Within 20 years the possibility of working with DNA at the molecular level had been realized. One of the most important steps was the development of recombinant deoxyribonucleic acid (rDNA) techniques. The rDNA technique involves the insertion of one piece of DNA into another, including between unrelated organisms. rDNA was immediately recognized to be an extremely powerful technology, and fears about its use soon emerged, leading to a temporary halt in rDNA experiments. The experiments restarted a couple of years later. The technology was soon applied to a range of new biotechnological products, including pharmaceuticals and transgenic organisms.

Chargraff had shown that the four bases of DNA, adenine, thymine, guanine, and cytosine, did not form a repetitive sequence and could therefore be capable of carrying the genetic code. It remained to be shown how this code functioned and how the information from the code could be transferred to enable the building of proteins. In 1957 it was suggested by Frances Crick and George Gamow that the genetic code referred to the sequence of the amino acids that make up proteins. There are 20 amino acids to code for and 4 bases to code for them. This meant that it was most likely for the bases to code for amino acids in groups of three because this would produce sufficient variations in the code. The bases separately could code for only 4 amino acids, in pairs for 16, while triplets gave 64 possibilities. The triplets of bases are referred to as codons.

Marshall Nirenberg made the first link between a codon and the amino acid it specified in 1961. This corresponded to an AAA codon on a strand of DNA and specified the amino acid lysine. Nirenberg's team had worked out the rest of the codon "dictionary" by 1966. In some cases two or more codons specify the same amino acid and three codons do not specify an amino acid but instead a point in the code at which translation (the reading and converting of the code) should stop—they are therefore referred to as stop codons.

It was known that DNA would have a replication mechanism, and the process of replication was observed in 1957. It was later discovered how ribonucleic acid (RNA) carried sections of the genetic code out of the nucleus to build proteins. RNA is similar to DNA, although it is normally single stranded and the base thymine of DNA is replaced by the base uracil (U) in RNA, so it has the bases A, U, G, and C. In studies of the cell, RNA had been shown to be present both in the nucleus and in the cytoplasm (the part of the cell surrounding the nucleus).

There are three types of RNA in cells, and each has a different function. The only one present in the nucleus of cells is messenger ribonucleic acid (mRNA), and it is this that carries the genetic code from the DNA out into the cytoplasm where the proteins are built. It was observed that certain sections of DNA will unravel temporarily and the mRNA will match up to one side of the strand and by matching the nucleotide bases A to T, U to A, C to G, and G to C can then carry the code away while the DNA rewinds. Back in the cytoplasm the mRNA is then translated into amino acids, which the transfer ribonucleic acid (tRNA) collects and the ribosomal ribonucleic acid (rRNA) builds into proteins.

The discovery of how genes code for proteins was an important step toward the development of rDNA techniques. Also important were the discovery of restriction enzymes and DNA ligase. Restriction enzymes can "cut" DNA at specific points in the base sequence and were discovered by Hamilton Smith and David Nathans in 1971. Viruses use such enzymes to insert their RNA into a host's DNA. DNA ligase is an enzyme that can "stick" two strands of DNA together. In 1972 the biochemist Paul Berg used a restriction enzyme to cut strands of DNA and used ligase to stick two strands together in a novel way. This created the first rDNA molecule.

With this new technique it became possible to transfer genetic information across species boundaries and to manipulate DNA in a controlled manner "to modify genes or to design new ones, to insert them into bacterial cells . . . and thus to form cells with new biochemical properties" (Asimov, 1987, p. 591). Concerns were soon raised within the scientific community about the safety of rDNA experiments, with particular fears about accidental release of genetically altered bacteria or viruses. This led to a halt in experiments following a discussion at the 1975 Asilomar Conference, until guidelines had been introduced. The US National Institutes of Health (NIH) issued guidelines the following year, and research continued. rDNA gave scientists "methods of participating directly in gene activity" (Asimov, 1987, p. 591), and the ability to create entirely new products from biological processes brought about many biotechnological applications.

Early examples include the production of human insulin (1978) and human growth hormone (first cloned in 1979), transgenic mice (1981), and later genetically modified crops (first field trials in 1985) and gene therapies (1990).

Genome Sequencing

Another important development in genetic engineering has been the sequencing of genomes. This developed from the early work of geneticists on locating and mapping genes on chromosomes. Current techniques and knowledge now allow much more sophisticated mapping to be done, and sequencing is a first step in the mapping process. Advances in sequencing tools, and particularly the increased speed at which the information produced can be processed, meant that it was possible to begin sequencing the human genome in 1990, and a full draft of the human genome was published in April 2003. Sequencing of genomes has greatly increased the amount of genetic information available to scientists, and this will, among other things, enable them to gain increased knowledge of human diseases—"When we have a detailed genetic map we will be able to identify whole sets of genes that influence general aspects of how the body grows or how the body fails to function" (Kevles and Hood, 1992, p. 94).

Mapping of genes is the "determination of the relative positions of genes on a DNA molecule (chromosome or plasmid) and of the distance, in linkage units or physical units, between them" (Kevles and Hood, 1992, p. 379). The first linkage or chromosome map was created by A. H. Sturtevant in 1913 and mapped the relative locations of six genes on one chromosome of *Drosophila*. Early mapping used mutations (genetic changes) to establish the location of genes on particular chromosomes. Mutations can be studied relatively easily in fruit flies as they breed rapidly, allowing genetic changes to be followed through many generations, but it was difficult to do this work on humans because their life cycle is far longer. A new technique, developed in 1967, changed this. Somatic cell hybridization enabled work to be done on mapping human genes. Somatic cell hybridization mixes chromosomes from human cells and mice cells, creating single cells containing both sets of chromosomes. These cells are not very stable, and as they divide human chromosomes are lost.

When only one human chromosome is left in the cell, any human proteins produced by the cell must be the expression of genes on that chromosome. Genetic sequencing determines the sequence of nucleotides (the individual nucleic acids adenine, thymine, guanine, and cytosine) present in a gene. Sequencing of genes did not become possible until the structure and role of DNA were understood. The development of the codon dictionary was particularly important to this.

Frederick Sanger began work on DNA sequencing in 1977, building on his previous work on establishing the sequence of amino acids in proteins. He completed the first genome sequence (of a bacteriophage named phiX174) in 1978. Another method of sequencing was developed at the same time, which used chemicals instead of dideoxynucleotides to split up the DNA. "Since then, the two methods have been standardized, speeded up and in a large part automated" (Kevles and Hood, 1992, p. 66). The development of the polymerase chain reaction (PCR) in 1980 by the Cetus Corporation helped to speed up the process of sequencing. PCR is a method of replicating fragments of DNA many times over, rapidly providing large amounts for analysis and sequencing. Computers helped both to automate the process and to store the vast data produced.

These developments made conceivable the sequencing of larger genomes, such as the human genome, the idea of which began to be discussed in the mid-1980s. In 1988 the US Congress approved the HGP, a massive, international public project to sequence and map the human genome, and work began in 1990. The human genome is far larger than any genome previously sequenced (to compare, phiX174 has 5,375 nucleotide bases; the human genome has approximately 3,000,000,000). An ambitious target for completion of the sequence in 15 years was set. The work on sequencing the human genome (only one part of the overall project) progressed slowly until a privately funded initiative was set up in competition, in May 1998. This made use of a different sequencing method and promised far quicker results for less money. This move was and still is hugely controversial but did spur on efforts within the public project. Both projects published rough drafts of the human genome in February 2001, and the public project released a full draft in April 2003.

The human genome sequence will provide the basis for detailed mapping of genes and their functions. One of the most direct benefits to come from sequencing of the human genome will be enhanced understanding and therefore improved treatment of many human diseases, but the information resulting from the HGP will have many other applications as well.

It is not only the human genome that has been sequenced but also key reference genomes such as the fruit fly, nematode worm, and common house mouse; over 1,200 other genomes have been completely sequenced (Genomes Online, 2009), most of them microbial. The fruit fly was sequenced by the private team prior to its work on the human genome, to show that the sequencing method worked, and the nematode worm was sequenced by the public project to serve as a reference genome.

The mouse genome will also serve as an important reference for the HGP as it "will allow researchers to gain insights into the function of many human genes because the mouse carries virtually the same set of genes as the human but can be used in laboratory research" (NIH, 2002). Sequencing of the genomes of other organisms has established that sequencing tools and techniques work and has provided important reference information, as well as giving an understanding of the particular organism involved. An offshoot of the HGP is the Microbial Genome Program, which will increase understanding of various microorganisms in order that they might be better utilized by humans in waste treatment and environmental management and so that disease-causing microbes can be more effectively targeted by drugs. Information on many other genome-sequencing projects can be found through websites such as the Genomes Online Database (http://www.genomesonline.org).

The sequencing and mapping of genomes have contributed to increased knowledge of the biological processes of various organisms and to an understanding of genetic functions. They provide vast amounts of data to which the tools of genetic engineering can be applied, in turn increasing the scope of biotechnology applications.

Biotechnology Applications

Humans have been making use of living organisms and biological processes for thousands of years; the earliest applications were probably in the production of food and drink products such as beer, bread, and cheese. Early applications made use of entirely natural processes and did not require any understanding of what these processes were. Some applications of modern biotechnology still use naturally occurring processes, which are now far better understood. Genetic engineering has been used to improve the understanding of biological processes and to improve them, and it has also been used to create new sources of particular products and completely novel products that have never before occurred in nature. Biotechnology is now applied across a huge range of industries, and there has been a great expansion in the scope of its applications since the development of rDNA techniques.

The present range of industrial sectors using biotechnology includes health care, food, mining, plastics, chemical, textiles, and waste treatment. It is also widely used in agriculture and animal husbandry. There are far too many applications for them all to be discussed here, but some of their uses within these sectors are briefly outlined.

- **Health care**: The earliest applications of rDNA were to address problems of human health, and the pharmaceutical industry is the area where modern biotechnology has had its biggest impacts so far. The first applications of rDNA were to produce bacteria to "manufacture" human proteins.

An early example of this was the adaptation of *Escherichia coli* (*E. coli*) bacteria to produce human insulin. Insulin for the treatment of diabetes had previously been sourced from animals. The human version is better suited to fulfill this function and the huge quantities necessary to treat the 220 million people worldwide that have the disease (World Health Organization, 2009) and can be produced more reliably. The license to market human insulin produced in bacteria was granted in 1982 (Biotechnology Industry Organization, 2002). There are currently products approved for the treatment of many diseases and disorders, including hemophilia, hepatitis, certain cancers, heart disease, anemia, cystic fibrosis, and epilepsy. Recombinant vaccines and new diagnostic tests have also been developed.

- **Agriculture**: Biotechnology has been applied to agriculture in a number of ways, to both plants and animals. In food crops genetic engineering has been used to transfer or create a number of desirable traits. These include increased yields, reduced need for inputs like pesticides and herbicides, and the production of plants with improved nutritional value for both human consumption and use in animal feed. Currently there are genetically modified crops being developed to produce other useful products such as pharmaceutical drugs, vaccines, blood-clotting factors, and chemicals for use in industrial processes (Union of Concerned Scientists, 2004). Animals have also been genetically engineered to enhance desirable traits and to act as "factories" for producing other useful products. For example, cows have been genetically engineered to produce some human proteins in their milk. Similar developments have occurred in aquaculture or fish farming, particularly with the aim of speeding up growth rates.

- **Food and beverages**: This is the area with the longest history of applications of biotechnology. Natural biological processes have traditionally been exploited in processes such as the fermentation of alcohol, bread making, and cheese making. Modern biotechnology is being used to increase the understanding of and improve these processes. Rennet, for example, used to be sourced from calves' stomachs but can now be produced in genetically engineered bacteria, which produces a cheese suitable for consumption by vegetarians. New uses and processes have also been developed, particularly as the properties of more yeasts and fungi have been discovered and exploited. Further examples of uses are in preservatives and flavorings.

- **Mining**: Modern biotechnology has enabled the replacement of chemical methods for extracting some mineral ores by biological ones, which are often more effective and create fewer unwanted by-products. Sometimes the bacteria used are entirely natural, although genetic analysis may have been used to work out the most suitable bacteria and the optimum conditions for them to work under. Other bacteria may be specifically designed to do this work.

- **Environmental management**: Biotechnology is extremely useful in the treatment of waste products since biological processes are involved in the degrading of all wastes. Biological processes are used by many industries to treat their waste products in order to reduce the amount of pollution they create. Biotechnology is also used in the general treatment of public wastewater and sewage. Scientists have also begun work on optimizing the action of bacteria in landfill sites to speed up processes of degradation. Bacteria can also be used as a method of cleaning up oil spills. Similar to the use of bacteria in mineral extraction, many of the current applications make use of naturally occurring processes that are now better understood and can therefore be more effectively applied.

There can also be genetic modification of the bacteria involved, for example, to enable them to work under specific conditions, and cloning can be used to create large amounts of either naturally occurring bacteria with specific traits or the custom-made versions. Biotechnology has a major role not only in the treatment of wastes and spillages but also in preventing environmental damage in the first place by creating more environmentally friendly production processes: "Biotechnology offers us many options for minimizing the environmental impact of manufacturing processes by decreasing energy use and replacing harsh chemicals with biodegradable molecules produced by living things" (Biotechnology Industry Organization, 2002). Biological processes are already replacing the use of some chemicals in industries such as the paper pulp and textiles industries.

The Industry

Modern biotechnology has been applied across a wide variety of long-established industries, and it has also led to the formation of its own industry. The biotechnology industry has developed rapidly since its origins in the mid-1970s. As the applications of modern biotechnology continue to increase on the basis of new scientific developments, so is the industry also likely to continue its expansion.

Over the past 30 years strong links have been developed between academia and industry in the biotechnology area, with commercial applications often coming directly from work in academic laboratories. From the mid-1970s onward many small biotechnology start-up companies were created, often concentrating on the development of products, which would subsequently be manufactured and marketed by larger, established companies. The first such company, Genentech, was created in 1976. Genentech's first commercially available product was cloned human insulin (Olson, 1986, p. 85). Over the next few years, scientists set up several other start-up companies. Genentech did not take its product to market itself but instead licensed production to the pharmaceutical giant Eli Lilly. This made sense because Genentech did not have the capacity to manufacture or resources to market the product, which Eli Lilly as an established pharmaceutical company had.

Following the success of the small companies, the established pharmaceutical companies moved into the area in the early 1980s, taking over small biotechnology companies or setting up their own biotechnology sectors. An example of such a company is GlaxoSmithKline, one of the world's largest pharmaceutical companies, which currently has several biotech products approved and on the market. Its first biotech product—a recombinant hepatitis B vaccine—received approval in 1989 (Biotechnology Industry Organization, 2002). More recently GlaxoSmithKline has moved into genomics to enhance its research and development processes (GlaxoSmithKline, n.d.). In the mid- to late 1980s other companies from the chemical and seed industries began to enter the biotechnology area, often consolidating into huge life science companies. A well-known example of such a company is Monsanto. Monsanto was formed as a chemical company in 1901 and soon expanded its range of products and bought out many other companies. Monsanto has had an agricultural division since 1960 and moved into biotechnology in 1989 (Monsanto, 2002a). Its first biotech product, POSILAC bovine somatotropin, designed to improve milk production in dairy herds, was approved in 1993 (Monsanto, 2002b). Since then Monsanto has had over 20 genetically modified crops approved (AGBIOS, 2010). From 1997 Monsanto became involved, through collaborations, in genomics research and merged with a large pharmaceutical company in 2000 to form the Pharmacia Corporation. (A new Monsanto company was established as a subsidiary of Pharmacia in 2000 and became a separate company in 2002, which focuses on agricultural biotechnology and genomics.) The industry is predominantly based in major industrialized countries and centers in Europe, Japan, and the United States.

Conclusion

Biotechnology, being the use of biological processes to create useful products, has a long history. Rapid scientific developments in the past few decades have produced a knowledge base and a set of tools and techniques that enable biological processes to be understood and controlled to an extent never before possible. This has created the biotechnology revolution. During the first half of the twentieth century knowledge from the scientific fields of chemistry and genetics combined to provide the basis for a revolution in the life sciences. Advances in genetic engineering since 1953, which have allowed the manipulation of life processes at a genetic level, have given modern biotechnology its central tools and techniques. The unprecedented nature of these advances—in particular the ability to transfer genetic material from one organism to another (including across species boundaries)—has given the new biotechnology its revolutionary effects. Modern biotechnology has incorporated genetic engineering to create transgenic plants and animals, novel pharmaceutical products, improved methods of waste treatment, and far more.

There has clearly been a revolution in the life sciences on the basis of a new understanding and knowledge of genetics and new tools and techniques to apply this knowledge.

References

AGBIOS (n.d.). *GM Database*, http://www.agbios.com/dbase.php (accessed March 9, 2010).

Aldridge, S. (1996). *The Thread of Life: The Story of Genes and Genetic Engineering*. Cambridge: Cambridge University Press.

Asimov, I. (1987). *Asimov's New Guide to Science*. Harmondsworth: Penguin.

Biotechnology Industry Organization (2002). *Guide to Biotechnology: Industrial and Environmental Applications*, http://www.bio.org/er/industrial.asp (accessed September 24, 2002).

Fruton, J. S. (1972). *Molecules and Life, Historical Essays on the Interplay of Chemistry and Biology*. New York, NY: Wiley Interscience.

Genomes Online (2009). *Genomes Online Database V.3.0*, http://www.genomesonline.org/gold.cgi (accessed October 15, 2009).

GlaxoSmithKline (n.d.). *Creating Medicines: Overview*, http://science.gsk.com/creating/creating_01.htm (accessed 15 October 2009).

Hershey, A. D., and Chase, M. (1952). Independent functions of viral protein and nucleic acid in growth of bacteriophage. *Journal of General Physiology*, 36(1), 39–56.

Hudson, J. (1992). *The History of Chemistry*. London: Macmillan.

Kevles, D. J., and Hood, L. (eds.) (1992). *The Code of Codes: Scientific and Social Issues in the Human Genome Project*. London: Harvard University Press.

Monsanto (2002a). *About Us, Our Heritage: Company Timeline/History*, http://www.monsanto.com/monsanto/layout/about_us/timeline/default.asp (accessed October 18, 2002).

Monsanto (2002b). *POSILAC 1 Step TM Bovine Somatotropin by Monsanto*, http://www.monsantodairy.com (accessed November 15, 2002).

National Institutes of Health (2002). *International Team of Researchers Assembles Draft Sequence of Mouse Genome*, http://www.nih.gov/news/pr/may2002/nhgri-06.htm (accessed October 16, 2002).

Olson, S. (1986). *Biotechnology: An Industry Comes of Age*. Washington, DC: National Academies Press.

Union of Concerned Scientists (2004). *Pharmaceutical and Industrial Crops: Questions and Answers about a Growing Concern*, http://www.ucsusa.org/food_and_agriculture/science_and_impacts/impacts_genetic_engineering/faqs-about-pharmaceutical-and.html (accessed October 15, 2009).

World Health Organization (2009). *Factsheet No. 312: Diabetes*, http://www.who.int/mediacentre/factsheets/fs312/en/index.html (accessed February 18, 2010).

Chapter 3

The "Vicious Cycle" of Obesity

Eduardo A. Nillni

Division of Endocrinology, Department of Medicine,
The Warren Alpert Medical School of Brown University/Rhode Island
Hospital, Providence, RI 02903, USA
Department of Molecular Biology, Cell Biology and Biochemistry,
Brown University, Providence, RI 02912, USA
eduardo_nillni@brown.edu

We are currently witnessing a worldwide pandemic of obesity, where there are approximately 700 million obese people worldwide and another 2 billion who are overweight, as defined by the World Health Organization. These categories are based on the body mass index (BMI) as an index of obesity, which is a measurement in meters squared of the relative percentages of fat and muscle mass in the human body measured in kilograms and then divided by height. According to the Public Health Surveillance Program (the ongoing systematic collection, analysis, and interpretation of outcome-specific data) from the Centers for Disease Control (CDC) during the past 20 years, there has been a dramatic increase in obesity in the United States and rates remain high. More than one-third of US adults

Creating Life from Life: Biotechnology and Science Fiction
Edited by Rosalyn W. Berne
Copyright © 2015 Pan Stanford Publishing Pte. Ltd.
ISBN 978-981-4463-58-4 (Hardcover), 978-981-4463-59-1 (eBook)
www.panstanford.com

(35.7%) and approximately 17% (or 12.5 million) of children and adolescents aged 2–19 years are obese. In 2008 alone, the medical costs associated with obesity were estimated at $147 billion; the medical costs for people who are obese were $1,429 higher than those of normal weight (as per the CDC). We are witnessing today more obese and overweight people on the planet than people suffering from malnutrition. Despite the great progress made in this field, our limited understanding of this condition has been disappointing. A better understanding of these mechanisms will help us to find novel therapeutic approaches for treating obesity.

Although obesity, a consequence of the modern lifestyle society, is not a disease per se, it has its severe side effects over time, causing a range of metabolic diseases, including type 2 diabetes and associated cardiovascular diseases, glucose intolerance, hyperlipidemia, and liver disease. These diseases have increased in pandemic proportions in the United States and in lesser degree in other countries, with no reversal despite educational programs and treatment options. These unsuccessful strategies are a consequence of a lack of knowledge about the precise pathology and etiology of metabolic disorders.

Definition of Obesity and Our Evolutionary Traits

Obesity and its related medical complications, including type 2 diabetes, cardiovascular disease, dyslipidemia, and cancer, account for more than 300,000 deaths per year in the United States. Obesity treatment strategies often do not result in adequate sustained weight loss, and the prevalence and severity of obesity in the United States and many developed countries is progressively increasing. Recent surveys classify roughly one-third of all Americans as obese. The complexity of the obesity condition results from the interaction between environmental and predisposed genetic factors. A more thorough understanding of the molecular mechanisms underlying the pathogenesis of obesity and the regulation of energy metabolism is essential for the development of effective therapies.

Obesity occurs as a result of a long-standing imbalance between energy intake and energy expenditure, which is influenced by a very complex set of biological pathway systems regulating appetite and a complex interaction between the environmental and genetic factors, while monogenic defects are relatively rare. A better understanding of the causes of obesity lies in uncovering the molecular and physiologic mechanisms that regulate appetite, satiety, and energy balance and will further improve the possibility to develop new antiobesity drugs.

Our Genetic Makeup over the Course of Evolution

The factors contributing to obesity in a society with unnatural access to calories and processed food are multiple and in great part due to an exacerbation of our evolutionary genes to promote survival. Genes enhancing obesity bring up an interesting observation, because obesity seems to cause with time a host of negative consequences. During the course of evolution by natural selection all species, including humans, develop genes through natural selection, which favors advantages in dealing with the environment, not disadvantages. Therefore, how is it possible for us to become an obese species if obesity is a negative trait that will threaten our survival and should have eliminated us as species? It is important to point out that similarly to humans many animals accumulate body fat in amounts that would be considered obesity in humans. The most typical examples are hibernating animals, which deposit enormous fat stores before entering hibernation, and migratory birds, which deposit similar stores before starting on migratory journeys. It is clear from these situations of temporary obesity as a mechanism of survival in anticipation of a future shortfall of energy. It will be catastrophic for hibernating animals to be unable to feed in winter and for migratory birds to be unable to feed enough before flying over oceans. A lack of genes favoring fat accumulation will exterminate these species. Primitive humans had the same evolutionary genes, which allowed them to survive during periods of starvation.

Lack of Respect for Evolutionary Traits by Modern Society: Changes in the Energy Balance Set Point

We could argue that an energy-dense diet, high in saturated fat and sugar, should cause weight gain and increased adiposity but can be easily reversed by a more natural regimen of foods and lower calorie intake. However, it appears that these diets, maintained long term, cause a profound change in the energy balance that does not result from a simple increase in energetic intake, particularly for those individuals who pass the 30 BMI mark. Diets containing long-chain saturated fats result in metabolic dysfunction with increased adiposity and body weight that are protected, so any subsequent weight loss through calorie restriction is difficult to maintain. The center regulating all these processes is the hypothalamus, located in the base of the brain. The hypothalamus regulates the energy balance by integrating the information from peripheral and neuronal hormone signals directly sensing a lack or the presence of nutrients. This mechanism regulates food intake and energy expenditure but also the consumption and partitioning of nutrients.

The profound changes seen in the energy balance controlled by the hypothalamus result in the loss of central leptin and insulin sensitivity, which perpetuates the development of both obesity and peripheral insulin insensitivity. This hypothalamic dysfunction causes changes in the set point between energy intake and energy expenditure, which is defended by the brain at any cost. Continuous ingestion of an excess of high-fat diet induces changes in the hypothalamus, which include an increase of oxidative stress; chronic atypical neuronal inflammation; endoplasmic reticulum (ER) stress; changes in neuronal cellular death, called apoptosis; and neuronal rewiring. A number of mechanisms have been proposed to be critical in perpetuating the effect of a high-fat diet on hypothalamic dysfunction, including reactive oxygen species, lipid metabolism, autophagy, and neuronal and synaptic plasticity. These hypothalamic changes induced by a high-fat diet linked to inflammation, ER stress, and autophagy defects increase the development of obesity.

Inflammation and ER Stress Changing the Biochemistry of the Brain

It is puzzling how the brain, or any endocrine system for that matter, with its numerous levels of compensatory responses to maintain normal homeostasis can be so easily compromised and disrupted in obesity. A key factor in the development of obesity across the human population is the availability of highly palatable, energy-dense foods high in saturated fats and refined sugars. Overnutrition over time is a contributory factor triggering a specific innate mechanism of the immune system and causing an atypical inflammation that is fundamental in the development of obesity and metabolic disease, as seen in humans with an increase in inflammatory markers in the circulation. Thus, it is now widely accepted that obesity is related to low levels of systemic inflammation.

Overnutrition is also responsible for the development of ER stress that occurs in the hypothalamus as well as in peripheral tissues. The ER is a compartment within the cell that produces proteins and hormones for secretion and for intracellular function essential for the biology of the cell and important in the communication among organs in all animals. When the demand for more anorexigenic (calorie-burning) hormones is high to keep coping with overnutrition a cellular stress is established. Obesity and dysregulation of appetite-regulating hormones have recently been linked to ER stress. When the ER becomes stressed because of an excessive accumulation of newly synthesized unfolded proteins, the unfolded protein response (UPR) is activated. These UPR pathways act in concert to increase ER content, expand the ER protein-folding capacity, degrade misfolded proteins, and reduce the load of new proteins entering the ER. This is an adaptive response geared toward resolving the protein-folding defect. Early studies showed that obesity-induced ER stress impairs insulin biosynthesis in pancreatic B cells by affecting pro-insulin folding, processing, and insulin release. In addition, hypothalamic ER stress has been proposed as one of the possible causes inducing leptin resistance and altered energy balance during obesity. The UPR enables the cell to manage the requirements for protein synthesis. If this process continues without control it can lead to apoptosis and cell death, as in the case of type 2 diabetes, where an increasing demand to produce insulin from the pancreatic B cells eventually leads to death. In the hypothalamus, the UPR results from a high-fat diet and has been shown to be both a cause and a consequence of inflammation. ER stress produced in the brain is also responsible for profound changes in the production of key hormones regulating the energy balance. A new discovery from our laboratory proves that point.

Our novel results using the obese model strongly suggests that obesity-induced ER stress obstructs the normal post-translational processing of pro-opiomelanocortin (POMC) causing less alpha–melanocyte-stimulating hormone (α-MSH) production, a strong anorexigenic hormone responsible for increasing energy expenditure. The root cause appears to be a breakdown in the protein-processing mechanism of the cells. These complex sets of neurochemical processes, newly unraveled in our laboratory, show that obesity can sustain itself, impeding hormones that would curb appetite or increase the burn rate for calories, a state we called a "vicious cycle," involving a breakdown of how the brain cells process key proteins, which allow obesity to beget further obesity. Although we knew before this study that one mechanism in which obesity perpetuates itself (as explained above) was by causing resistance to leptin, a hormone that signals the brain about the status of fat in the body, we know now that there is much more than just leptin resistance. α-MSH has two jobs in parts of the hypothalamus region of the brain. One is to suppress the activity of food-seeking-behavior brain cells. The second is to signal other brain cells to produce the hormone thyroid-regulating hormone (TRH), which prompts the thyroid gland to spur calorie-burning activity in the body.

In obese rats α-MSH was low despite an abundance of leptin and despite normal levels of gene expression both for its biochemical precursor protein called POMC and for a key enzyme called PC2, which processes POMC in brain cells. There had to be more to the story than just leptin. In our studies we found out where the α-MSH deficit was coming from: a disruption in the mechanism for processing POMC to make α-MSH.

Protein-Processing Problems

We subjected a group of rats to a high-calorie diet and others to a normal diet for 12 weeks. The overfed rats developed a condition of "diet-induced obesity." Then we studied the hormone levels and brain cell physiology of the rats. We found that in the obese rats, a key "machine" in the brain cells' assembly line of protein making, called the ER, becomes stressed and overwhelmed. The overloaded ER apparently fumbles the proper handling of the enzyme PC2, perhaps discarding it because it can't be folded up properly. The PC2 levels we measured in obese rats, for example, were 53% lower than in normal rats. α-MSH peptides were also barely more than half as abundant in obese rats as they were in healthy rats. In our study we showed that what actually prevents the production of more α-MSH peptide is that ER stress was decreasing the biosynthesis of POMC by affecting one key enzyme that is essential for the formation of α-MSH, a totally novel mechanism.

We confirmed our findings in several ways: In obese rats we measured elevated levels of known markers of ER stress. We also purposely induced ER stress in cells using pharmacological agents and saw that both PC2 and α-MSH levels dropped. Next we conducted an experiment to see if fixing ER stress would improve α-MSH production. We treated lean and obese rats for two days with a chemical called TUDCA, which is known to alleviate ER stress. If ER stress was responsible for α-MSH production problems, we would see α-MSH recover in obese rats treated with TUDCA. Sure enough, while TUDCA didn't increase α-MSH production in the lean rats, it increased it markedly in the obese rats. Similarly on the bench top we took mouse neurons that produce PC2 and POMC and pretreated some with a similar chemical called PBA, which prevents ER stress. We left others untreated. Then we induced ER stress in all the cells. Under that ER stress, those that had been pretreated with PBA produced about twice as much PC2 as those that had not.

A word of caution is that although we found ways to restore PC2 and α-MSH by treating ER stress in living rats and individual cells, the agents used in the study are not readily applicable as medicines for treating obesity in humans, because they are not approved by the Food and Drug Administration (FDA) in the present form. But by laying out the exact mechanism responsible for why the brains of obese rats failed to curb appetite or spur greater calorie burning, the present study points drug makers to several opportunities where they can intervene to break this new, vicious cycle that helps obesity to perpetuate itself. Understanding the central control of energy-regulating neuropeptides during diet-induced obesity is important for the identification of therapeutic targets to prevent and/or mitigate obesity pathology. Taken together, overnutrition can damage the neuronal substrate of the energy balance at many levels ranging from the intracellular to the structure of key neuronal interactions, thus contributing to obesity and metabolic dysfunction. Importantly these mechanisms are only now beginning to be characterized, and in doing so many potential drug targets may be revealed to combat obesity and related diseases.

Acknowledgments

This was supported by the National Institute of Diabetes and Digestive and Kidney Diseases/National Institutes of Health Grant 5R01 DK085916-04 and 3R01 DK085916-03S1.

Madeline

Rosalyn W. Berne

MADELINE SAT WHERE SHE always sat whenever the weather was amenable. She favored the wooden bench painted in a high-gloss green, secured by bolts into the concrete, although the effort it took to get there was exhausting: down two flights of stairs, through the heavy steel door, out onto the shrub-lined, bricked walkway between buildings 111 and 113, and into the interior courtyard. Once she was there, and settled in, the thought of going back home became daunting.

On most days, when the sky was blue and the sun was bright, she'd sit watching the children play. Madeline, like the bench on which she sat, the slick sliding board, galvanized jungle gym, and painted wooden seesaw, was a fixture in the community courtyard—a fixture, though she moved, to an extent, and breathed, but with great effort, and smiled readily through her ruddy red cheeks, with pink lips made taut when upturned.

The design was intended to encourage human interaction, so that residents would be inclined to spend time out in the interior yard of the historic space. A century ago, when functioning as a factory, these brick buildings were filled with stitching machines and huge spools of thread, barrels of tannins, and animal hides. Now they had buffed heart pine floors, high painted ceilings, brightly colored entries, tile baths and cozy bedrooms, skylights and roof top gardens. Where shipping cartons were once stored on crates under tarps, there were now rose bushes and irises, water features, walkways, a tot-lot with a sandbox, and a playground, placed among the many trees.

Madeline had come to Philadelphia from Greece, arriving as Magdaliní, thankful for the wonders of her new life. Here she could live well, better than there, especially with the support of the Foundation. The Foundation considered her condition a disability, one that was no fault of her own. Its charter was to help those who, like her, were obese to the detriment of society. It's not as if she ate too much. At least she didn't think so. Her body was simply and innocently huge, exceeding the capacity of a normal desk chair or bus seat, and too big for the standing work of a store clerk or theater ticket taker. The weight increased incrementally over the years, until there was little she could do for herself other than to sit, sleep, and eat. To bathe, dress, and do her hair all involved significant strain.

Outside, beyond the wrought-iron gates leading from the community into the city, Madeline was no longer welcome, such an atrocity as she was. In her younger days, her lighter days, and before the ordinance against obesity, Madeline would spend mornings strolling through the Museum of Art and afternoons exploring the stacks of the Philadelphia Public Library. Sometimes her happy excursions became diversions, and Madeline would find herself south of the Liberty Bell, all the way down Ninth Street at the Italian Market. There she would delight in thumping melons; sniffing fresh thyme, oregano, and rosemary; and taking the firm roundness of orange, yellow, and green citruses into her hands, squeezing them ever so gently. Madeline enjoyed a nice ripe cheese, a thick slice of salami, an olive-oiled pasta as much as anyone but not more. There was nothing unusual about her appetite. It'd been years since she'd left to walk to a store or take a train to Center City. Getting to the bench was her daily conquest.

Madeline, supplied with a lunch and three snacks, sat alone on her bench in the community yard on sunny days, cloudy days, and hot and cold days, too. She would sit doing handiwork, knitting, crochet, and needlepoint, though her plump fingers could barely manipulate the needles anymore.

One weekend morning a girl called Bobbie sat down on the playground bench next to Madeline, which was delightful because the children rarely sat beside her. She reached over her knees to retie her loose laces. "Laces have a way of coming undone no matter how well you tie them," Madeline offered, aiming to reassure the child. The comment, well meant, was met with a blank stare.

"I bet you couldn't tie your own laces," Bobbie returned.

"Probably not," Madeline answered, knowing full well she definitely couldn't, which is why all her shoes were the slip-on kind.

"Why do you smell that way?" the child asked as she rose to her feet, crossing her arms over her chest.

"What way?" Madeline asked.

"Sour, sort of like eggs in vinegar."

Madeline considered Bobbie's query, for which she had no direct response. *Everyone has a scent, don't they? Perhaps some of us are more pungent than others.*

"Am I bothering you, my dear?" she asked.

The child shrugged and returned to her play, tossing a stone into the stretch of squares and rectangles below her and hopping on one foot and then the other, her aim to stay within the white demarcation lines. Suddenly the girl stopped, one foot in square 6 and the other in square 7, huffing and puffing from frustration. "Don't give up. You can do it!" Madeline offered. The child, joined by two others in her play, acted as if Madeline had not spoken.

A few weeks later, under the bright sun of a lovely Wednesday morning, Madeline was detained in the Italian Market. Two Foundation agents took her aside. The first words she spoke as they issued the decree were, "But why?" She couldn't help that her body was like her mother's, and like her grandmother's, too.

"Step onto the scale," they instructed.

Her heart raced as she anticipated the results. Rarely did she eat more meals than the Foundation allotted, or consumed more than the specified amount of food. (Perhaps once in a while she got hungry and did.) It wasn't as if she didn't weigh in occasionally to be sure she was within the limits. The problem was that the weight management center was five blocks past the cathedral (the one with the gold-domed roof and Venetian glass tiles that reminded her so much of home). Given how slowly she moved, and the nature of the neighborhood, the risk of being accosted again was too high. The last time she ventured there everything went well, her weight being under the maximum allowed. But on her way back home two boys and a girl accosted her and pulled her favorite blue shoes right off her feet. Thankfully someone saw the incident and called the Foundation hotline. She was treated for minor injuries and emotional trauma and then escorted directly to Unit 111.

On that particular day, at the Italian Market, Madeline did as she was told. She stepped onto the metal plate placed before her as a crowd gathered silently. The reading was plain for all to see, and it was a number she'd never expected. "You may step off the scale now," the agent directed. "I need to get one further reading."

He placed a small device against her biceps, transmitting the infrared light. The observers sounded an incredulous gasp as the ratio of her body fat was revealed.

"Oh my, 58!" one of the agents exclaimed.

An adolescent boy spoke out from the crowd adding, "And she stinks, too!"

Softly, in a whisper, Madeline asked the man if he noticed an odor. What he told Madeline, as he escorted her away was that, in fact, yes, she definitely reeked.

Forbidden back into the public sphere Madeline conspired spending her waking hours observing her residential community. One fall morning, while on her bench, crocheting a vest, she looked up to discover a group of adolescent boys encircling a teenaged girl. They lifted the girl's shirt and pointed to the roll of fat on her stomach, scolding her angrily. The girl hung her head and apologized. Madeline told the boys they should be ashamed of themselves, to which they raucously laughed, "But why?"

Late that afternoon, after a seven-hour stretch, Madeline stood from the bench. Slowly she strolled from one garden plot to another, noticing the asters, coneflowers, and black-eyed Susans in bloom. She noticed the branches of the trees lining the courtyard and how only few leaves remained—red ones here, yellow ones there, the ones above her head mostly brown and clinging with little strength remaining. She studied the bark of the sycamore tree, which grew from the center of the great community garden—how irregular were its patchy grays and beiges, shaped in seemingly random patterns.

Suddenly her knees were unable to hold her. It was a searing pain behind her left kneecap, which caused her to buckle under. As she lay there on the ground for nearly an hour, immobile, she noticed the changing pink and orange streaks across the sky, the pale green leafs sprouting on the branches, and the ant that crawled across her nose. There was nothing else she could do except cry.

Someone finally happened by and noticed Madeline, referring to her as "a heap of fat, bones, and flesh in a pile on the ground" while he made a call for help. The Foundation team came quickly, sedating her and then taking her away.

There was a time the Foundation might have used suction, stomach stapling, or stomach replacement to remove the fat, treating the effect rather than the actual cause. New methods were worth exploring. As a ward of the Foundation Madeline was given no choice. But of course she would receive the best of care. The procedure worked quite well on rats. Human trials could now begin. The cells, extracted from the cord of one never to be born, were injected into Madeline's tissues early the next morning.

Madeline remained indoors as winter passed, exercising, reading, and doing handiwork. Day by day her body released the fat, and week by week her weight diminished, though she worried that her vision grew more and more distorted, as if gel had been smeared across her eyes.

When finally spring arrived, bringing the sounds and scents of new life, Madeline felt drawn outside again. She returned to the community courtyard, no longer encumbered by excessive weight, yet she was very tired. Bobbie, Kaki, Shawna, and the other children at play wondered who this stranger might be. Madeline took a seat on the painted green bench to observe the children at play, smiling and waving to them. They looked up at her but said nothing, continuing on with their games.

Immersed in attentiveness to her fingertips, feeling across the stitches knit, Madeline was startled by the sound of an unfamiliar voice by her side. She'd not noticed when he sat down beside her.

"What are you making?" the unfamiliar man asked.

"Another sweater. I just don't know for whom."

He explained about being a newcomer to the neighborhood and how he'd read about the gardens and the courtyard, as described in the community spring newsletter. "I really like it here," he admitted, as he told her of his origins. He'd come from North Carolina to take a position at the nearby university.

Maybe it was the sound of his voice, its gentle tone, and soothing timbre. Madeline really liked him, even though they had only just met. Rarely did anyone ever speak to her, other than the children. So perhaps it was just his attention on her, but then again, maybe not. The pleasure of his company was visceral, though a reminder of how lonely she'd been.

"Really? A professor? And what is your field?"

Madeline leaned back a bit as he answered, trying to make out the expression on the man's face. He seemed genuinely engaged and jovial and maybe even interested in her. But she couldn't tell whether he was smiling or grimacing as he explained to her the subject matter of his research. She could see his forehead, at least most of it, and the fine lines around his eyes. But only part of his nose was discernable. And in the place where his lips might otherwise have been, was an oddly shaped blotch of dark gray.

There was no point in worrying, now was there? She could use her other senses to compensate. Any other strategy would be useless. So Madeline chose to adapt. After all, life was good. She felt mostly well. Aside from the fatigue, and the thirst, she definitely felt better than when she carried those extra 130 pounds. There was no need for alarm and nothing she need do.

"Fascinating," she said, not wanting to let on to the man how confusing it was to look at him. She must rely on her other senses, including her intuition.

I definitely like this man.

She noticed the lightness of her own being and the ease with which she was breathing, feeling gratitude for the beauty of the day. She considered the presence of the cells of another, established deeply in her own gray matter to provide the hormones she needed. It was with a refreshingly new perspective on life that she gazed across her surroundings, into a world she did not quite recognize as her own.

Chapter 4

Prion Diseases

Joel A. Pedersen

Univeristy of Wisconsin, 1525 Observatory Drive, Madison,
WI 53706, USA

joelpedersen@wisc.edu

Prion diseases, or transmissible spongiform encephalopathies (TSEs), are a family of insidious brain-wasting diseases that infect humans and other mammals. Human prion diseases include kuru, Creutzfeldt–Jakob disease (CJD), Gerstmann–Sträussler–Scheinker (GSS) disease, and fatal insomnia (FI). Prion diseases in nonhuman mammals include bovine spongiform encephalopathy (BSE), or "mad cow" disease, in cattle, chronic wasting disease (CWD) in North American members of the deer family, scrapie in sheep and goats, and transmissible mink encephalopathy (TME) in farmed mink. Prion diseases are characterized by a long incubation period (years to decades in humans) during which the infected individual does not display symptoms. Once clinical symptoms manifest, the disease progresses inexorably to death, often within six months. Prion disease symptoms in humans include dementia, memory loss, speech impairment, loss of motor control, personality changes, hallucinations, and

Creating Life from Life: Biotechnology and Science Fiction
Edited by Rosalyn W. Berne
Copyright © 2015 Pan Stanford Publishing Pte. Ltd.
ISBN 978-981-4463-58-4 (Hardcover), 978-981-4463-59-1 (eBook)
www.panstanford.com

seizures. The brains of infected individuals are characterized by the death of nerve cells, leading to a spongy appearance (hence "spongiform" encephalopathies) and accumulation of an abnormally folded form of the prion protein (PrP).

Prion diseases are caused by an enigmatic infectious agent that, unlike all other known pathogens, lacks genetic material (i.e., DNA, RNA). The infectious agent in these diseases is referred to as the prion and is composed primarily, if not solely, of misfolded forms of a normal cell surface protein. The normal form of the protein (denoted by PrP^C, where "C" is for cellular) is produced in many tissues throughout the body but especially in the nervous system. Disease-associated forms of the PrP are denoted by PrP^{TSE} (Brown and Cervenakova, 2005). Unlike bacterial pathogens, prions are not alive; unlike viruses they do not induce cells to make new infectious proteins from scratch. Instead, PrP^{TSE} promotes the misfolding of pre-existing PrP^C to the disease-associated state. During the preclinical and clinical phases of prion diseases, prions are present in the nervous system as well as the bloodstream and, in at least some species, are excreted in feces, urine, and saliva.

Prions are notoriously resistant to sterilization methods that are effective against conventional pathogens (e.g., bacteria, viruses, fungi). They withstand autoclaving under conditions typically used to sterilize medical equipment (Taylor, 2000). Boiling, treatment with alcohol, formaldehyde, or protein-degrading enzymes and irradiation with ultraviolet light, microwaves, or ionizing radiation have little effect on the infectious agent (Taylor, 2000). Remarkably, even incineration at 600°C (1080°F) for 15 minutes has been reported to not completely eliminate prion infectivity (Brown et al., 2004). Prions survive wastewater treatment (Hinckley et al., 2008) and can persist in the environment for years (Brown and Gajdusek, 1991; Seidel et al., 2007).

At present, diagnosis of prion diseases before clinical symptoms manifest is difficult because well-established detection methods lack the sensitivity necessary to detect prions in body fluids (e.g., blood, urine, cerebrospinal fluid). A number of experimental detection methods under development hold promise for early detection of prion diseases (e.g., Edgeworth et al., 2011; Saá, Castilla, and Soto, 2006; Sano et al., 2013). No cure is available for prion diseases once symptoms manifest.

Natural Transmission of Prion Diseases

Scrapie and chronic wasting disease (CWD) are unique among prion diseases in that they are transmitted among individuals by either direct (animal-to-animal) or indirect (animal–environment–animal) routes. Transmission of this nature is referred to as horizontal transmission to distinguish it from transmission via the food chain (vertical transmission). The shedding of prions in secretions and excreta of infected individuals facilitates horizontal transmission. Vertical transmission is due to the presence of prions in ingested material (e.g., the framed mink apparently acquiring transmissible mink encephalopathy [TME] from consuming the meat of downer cattle). The remarkable stability of prions leads to their persistence in the environment (Brown and Gajdusek, 1991; Seidel et al., 2007). Environmental transmission of scrapie has been recognized for centuries (Schneider, Fangerau, Michaelsen, and Raab, 2008), shepherds believing that scrapie-contaminated pastures were cursed. Indirect transmission of CWD has been demonstrated in captive deer facilities (Miller et al., 2004) and may contribute to the spread of the disease among wild deer, elk, and moose (Pedersen and Somerville, 2012). At the time of writing, CWD had been reported in free-ranging or captive deer and elk from 22 US states, two Canadian provinces, and South Korea. The disease is spreading unchecked among wild deer and elk in North America.

Human prion diseases arise via three routes: exposure to prions from outside the host (infectious prion disease), mutation in germ cells (sperm or egg cells), and, apparently, spontaneous misfolding or mutation in somatic cells (cells other than germ cells; e.g., sporadic Creutzfeldt–Jakob disease [sCJD]) (Colby and Prusiner, 2011; Watts, Balachandran, and Westaway, 2006). We are remarkably fortunate that human prion diseases are not spread horizontally. If CJD spread as easily as CWD transmits among deer, we would face a prion disease crisis of global proportions. Nevertheless, prion diseases have been transmitted to humans via ingestion of infected tissue and due to medical procedures.

The only known epidemic of purely human prion disease resulted from vertical transmission. The Fore tribe and adjacent linguistic groups in the New Guinea highlands experienced an epidemic of the prion disease kuru (from the Fore word "to shake") during the twentieth century (Gajdusek, 1977). The disease was transmitted through ritualistic endocannibalism: family members consumed their dead relatives in mortuary feasts (Manuelidis, Chakrabarty, Miyazawa, Nduom, and Emmerling, 2009). The incidence of kuru declined rapidly after Australian authorities prohibited the practice of cannibalism in the 1950s. The few cases reported during the first decade of the twenty-first century indicate that the incubation period can exceed 50 years (Collinge et al., 2006).

Transmission of Prion Diseases Assisted by Technology

Animal processing and medical technologies have contributed to the transmission of nonhuman and human prion diseases. In the late 1970s and early 1980s, changes in rendering technology (lower sterilization temperatures and omission of a solvent extraction step) in the U.K. resulted in prions not being excluded from bovine meat and bone meal (Nathanson, Wilesmith, and Griot, 1997). This product was fed to cattle as a protein supplement in an industrialized form of cannibalism, leading to the recycling of bovine spongiform encephalopathy (BSE) prions in the bovine food chain. BSE was initially identified in cattle in

1985 and resulted in an epidemic with more than 180,000 clinical cases in U.K. cattle (Ironside, 2012). Not all infected cattle would have shown clinical symptoms at the time of slaughter. The total number of cattle infected (symptomatic and asymptomatic) may be as high as 3 million (Ironside, 2012). Many of these cattle entered the human food supply. Prion-contaminated meat and bone meal were exported to other European countries, expanding the epidemic geographically (Nathanson et al., 1997). Outside Europe, BSE cases have been reported in the U.S., Canada, Japan, and Brazil. Multiple stains of BSE prions have been identified.

CJD has been transmitted through a variety of medical procedures that unknowingly exposed individuals to hormones, neural tissue, or eye tissue from individuals with undiagnosed sCJD infections. Such cases are referred to as iatrogenic CJD. The largest numbers of cases were due to grafts of dura mater, a membrane that envelops the brain (228 cases), and from human growth hormone derived from cadavers infected with sCJD (at least 226 cases) (Brown et al., 2012). Smaller numbers of cases were due to neurosurgery with contaminated instruments (2 cases), corneal transplants (at least 2 cases), and treatment with cadaver-derived pituitary hormone (gonadotropin) (4 cases) (Brown et al., 2012). Incubation periods in iatrogenic CJD ranged from 1 to 42 years. Pharmaceuticals derived from human body fluids may pose a risk of iatrogenic CJD transmission if infected individuals are not excluded from donor pools and prions copurify with the desired active component(s).

Urine-derived gonadotropins prescribed to treat infertility serve to illustrate the potential risk. More than 300,000 women in North America are treated with urine-derived gonadotropin annually (Van Dorsselaer et al., 2011). Research on laboratory animals has demonstrated that PrP^{TSE} can be excreted in urine (Kariv-Inbal, Ben-Hur, Grigoriadis, Engelstein, and Gabizon, 2006; Seeger et al., 2005), and the noninfectious form of PrP has been found as a contaminant in injectable fertility products derived from urine (Van Dorsselaer et al., 2011). The urine used to derive such products is obtained from thousands of donors through a system that does not currently permit donor tracing. At present, preclinical diagnosis of sCJD is not possible using a blood-screening test. Prevention of new cases of iatrogenic CJD currently relies on recognizing potentially infected individuals and employing new disinfection methods for biological products and delicate surgical instruments (Brown et al., 2012).

Interspecies Transmission to Humans: The Case of BSE

A curious feature of prions, given their composition, is the existence of strains differing in their virulence, clinical symptoms, and tissue distribution of PrP^{TSE}. Some prion strains have crossed into new host species and acquired new strain characteristics in a process referred to as adaptation. Prions that have adapted to a new host can exhibit an altered host range (Bartz, Marsh, McKenzie, and Aiken, 1998). For example, CWD prions from mule deer were able to infect ferrets but not hamsters. After several disease cycles in ferrets ("serial passage"), the new ferret-adapted strain could infect hamsters.

The transmission of BSE to humans in the form of variant Creutzfeldt–Jakob disease (vCJD) represents the only demonstrated case of interspecies transmission of a prion disease to humans. In 1996, epidemiological surveillance for CJD in the U.K. identified a new variant form of CJD (Will et al., 1996). The disease was recognized as distinct from sCJD because vCJD victims were much younger and showed different disease signs. Epidemiological and experimental evidence linked the emergence of vCJD to BSE (Ironside, 2012). Consumption of infected meat products was indicated as the most likely main route of human exposure to the BSE agent (Ward et al., 2006). As of February 2012, 176 confirmed and probable cases of vCJD in the U.K. and 49 cases in 11 other countries had been reported (Ironside, 2012). The estimated incubation period for the cases that have manifested so far is 17 years, and the median duration from onset of symptoms to death is 13 to 14 months (Holman et al., 2010). Contaminated feed also led to the transmission of BSE to domestic cats and captive wild cats (five species), antelope (six species), bison, lemurs (three species), and monkeys.

Since 1999–2000, the number of new vCJD cases per year has decreased in the U.K., and no patients with vCJD are alive at present (Ironside, 2012). The amino acid residue coded for at position 129 of the PrP gene strongly influences an individual's susceptibility to prion infection and the length of the incubation period (Cervenakova et al., 1998; Collinge, Palmer, and Dryden, 1991; Palmer, Dryden, Hughes, and Collinge, 1991). Individuals carry two copies of the PrP gene, each of which can code for either methionine (M) or valine (V) at position 129. A person can therefore have both copies coding for M (MM homozygous), both copies coding for V (VV homozygous), or one copy coding for each of M and V (MV heterozygous). The frequency of these variants at position 129 in Caucasians is 37% MM, 51% MV, and 12% VV (Collinge et al., 1991). Examination of archived tonsil and appendix samples in the U.K. suggests that approximately 1 in 10,000 individuals is an asymptomatic carrier of the disease (Clewley et al., 2009; Hilton et al., 2004); with only one exception all symptomatic individuals with vCJD were MM homozygotes (Ironside, 2012; Kaski et al., 2009). Some of the asymptomatic individuals who were positive for vCJD in their tonsil or appendix tissues were MV heterozygotes or VV homozygotes, indicating these genotypes can become infected and may have longer incubation periods than MM homozygotes (Clewley et al., 2009; Hilton et al., 2004; Ironside et al., 2006). These results may portend additional waves of vCJD cases in individuals who are not MM homozygotes, following longer incubation periods.

The existence of asymptomatic carriers of vCJD raises the specter of possible iatrogenic transmission with the possibility of further adaptation of vCJD prions to their human hosts. Indeed, secondary transmission of vCJD through contaminated blood products has already occurred. Three individuals in the U.K. who received packed red blood cells from asymptomatic donors who later died from vCJD have contracted the disease (Brown et al., 2012). All three recipients were MM homozygotes (Ironside, 2012). Incubation periods were 6.5 to 7.8 years (Ironside, 2012). Postmortem examination of a fourth individual (a MV heterozygote) who had received contaminated plasma products but was asymptomatic at death indicated infection with vCJD. Given the current difficulties in detecting asymptomatic human prion disease and the number of asymptomatic individuals, concern exists that the safety of the blood supply may be compromised in the U.K. and other countries that experienced BSE outbreaks. Recycling of vCJD prions in the human blood supply provides a means to serially passage the agent in human hosts. This could lead to further adaption of the agent to humans and lead to the emergence of a more virulent form of vCJD, possibly with altered disease symptoms.

Transmission of CWD to Humans: A Cause for Concern?

CWD affects North American members of the deer family, including elk, mule deer, white-tailed deer, and moose. The dramatic spread of the known range of CWD in North America since 2000 has raised concerns about the risk of transmission of this disease to humans through consumption of infected venison. No cases of human prion disease have been linked to CWD to date (Anderson et al., 2007; Belay et al., 2004; Mawhinney et al., 2006), and available experimental data suggests that a barrier exists to transmission to humans. Transmission of CWD to two nonhuman primates has been examined (Race et al., 2009). Squirrel monkeys were found to be susceptible to CWD by both intracerebral and oral routes of exposure, developing a severe wasting syndrome. In contrast, macaques, which are considered evolutionarily closer to humans, did not acquire clinical prion disease at 70 months postinoculation. Whether macaques can acquire subclinical CWD infection (and therefore serve as carriers of the disease) is unknown at present. CWD fails to transmit to mice genetically engineered to express human PrP (Kong et al., 2005; Sandberg et al., 2010; Tamgüney et al., 2006; Wilson et al., 2012). In an in vitro assay, a CWD agent converts human cellular prion protein (PrP^C) much less efficiently than does a classical BSE agent, suggesting a lower risk of cross-species transmission and also that the transmission barrier may not be absolute (Barria et al., 2014).

Uncertainty remains about the potential for CWD to transmit to humans. The existence of multiple CWD strains is recognized (Angers et al., 2010), but how many are present in infected deer, elk, and moose across North America is unknown. Prion strains can change within species as well as upon transmission to a new host species (Sandberg et al., 2010). Prion strains may differ in their ability to transmit disease to humans, and this ability may be affected by the genotype of the individuals exposed to the disease agent. The public health risk associated with CWD may depend on both the prion strain and the PrP genotype of the host. The lack of increase in recognizable prion diseases in areas where CWD is prevalent is comforting, but if CWD manifests as a wasting syndrome in humans similar to that observed in CWD-infected squirrel monkeys (Race et al., 2009), the disease may be misdiagnosed as a metabolic disorder and patients may never be tested for prion disease. Indeed, if vCJD victims had not been much younger than those of other forms of CJD, this disease may never have been identified. Human exposure to CWD prions is occurring and is likely to increase as the geographical range of the disease expands into more densely populated regions. Some hunters and their families knowingly consume CWD-infected venison. Others are exposed unwittingly. For example, 81 individuals unknowingly consumed or were exposed to a CWD-positive deer donated to a rural game feast in upstate New York (Garruto et al., 2008). Given the experience with vCJD, the possibility that humans may acquire subclinical CWD infection must also be considered. Subclinical infection could lead to transmission by blood transfusion or other medical procedures. Such transmission might allow CWD prions an opportunity to adapt to their new human host.

Transmission of Other Protein-Misfolding Diseases

Misfolded proteins figure prominently in a number of other diseases, including Alzheimer's disease, type 2 diabetes, Parkinson's disease, Huntington's disease, and tauopathies. The molecular mechanisms of protein misfolding in these diseases are similar (Soto, 2012). While epidemiological evidence for the transmissibility of these diseases among humans is currently lacking, recent research has demonstrated that they can be transmitted experimentally (Clavaguera et al., 2013; Colby and Prusiner, 2011; Soto, 2012). Animal-to-animal transmission of disease by miniscule aggregates of misfolded protein has been demonstrated in two animal-protein-misfolding diseases: mouse senile amyloidosis (Xing et al., 2001) and amyloid-A amyloidosis in captive cheetahs (Zhang et al., 2008). Determining whether additional protein-misfolding diseases can be transmitted between individuals warrants further research.

Acknowledgments

Financial support from the National Science Foundation through CAREER grant CBET-0547484 and the National Institutes of Health through R01 NS060034 is gratefully acknowledged. I thank Chris J. Johnson for his helpful comments on an earlier version of this essay.

References

Anderson, C. A., Bosque, P., Filley, C. M., Arciniegas, D.B., Kleinschmidt-Demasters, B. K., Pape, W. J., . . . and Tyler, K. L. (2007). Colorado surveillance program for chronic wasting disease transmission to humans: lessons from 2 highly suspicious but negative cases. *Archives of Neurology*, 64, 439–441. doi:10.1001/archneur.64.3.439.

Angers, R. C., Kang, H. E., Napier, D., Browning, S., Seward, T., Mathiason, C., . . . and Telling, G. T. (2010). Prion strain mutation determined by prion protein conformational compatibility and primary structure. *Science*, 328, 1154–1158. doi:10.1126/science.1187107.

Barria, M. A., Balachandran, A., Morita, M., Kitamoto, T., Barron, R., Manson, J., . . . and Head, M. W. (2014). Molecular barriers to zoonotic transmission of prions. *Emerging Infectious Diseases*, 20, 88–97. doi:10.3201/eid2001.130858.

Bartz, J. C., Marsh, R. F., McKenzie, D., and Aiken, J. M. (1998). The host range of chronic wasting disease is altered on passage in ferrets. *Journal of General Virology*, 251, 297–301. doi:10.1006/viro.1998.9427.

Belay, E. D., Maddox, R. A., Williams, E. S., Miller, M. W., Gambetti, P., and Schonberger, L. B. (2004). Chronic wasting disease and potential transmission to humans. *Emerging Infectious Diseases*, 10, 977–984. doi:10.3201/eid0905.020577.

Brown, P., Brandel, J.-P., Sato, T., Nakamura, Y., MacKenzie, J., Will, R. G., . . . and Schonberger, L. B. (2012). Iatrogenic Creutzfeldt-Jakob disease, final assessment. *Emerging Infectious Diseases*, 18, 901–907. doi:10.3201/eid1806.120116.

Brown, P., and Cervenakova, L. (2005). A prion lexicon (out of control). *Lancet*, 365, 122.

Brown, P., and Gajdusek, D. C. (1991). Survival of scrapie virus after 3 years' interment. *Lancet*, 337, 269–270. doi:10.1016/0140-6736(91)90873-N.

Brown, P., Rau, E. H., Lemieux, P., Johnson, B. K., Bacote, A.E., and Gajdusek, D.C. (2004). Infectivity studies of both ash and air emissions from simulated incineration of scrapie-contaminated tissues. *Environmental Science & Technology*, 38, 6155–6160. doi:10.1021/es040301z.

Cervenakova, Goldfarb, L. G., Garruto, R., Lee, H. S., Gajdusek, D. C., and Brown, P. (1998). Phenotype-genotype studies in kuru: implications for new variant Creutzfeldt-Jakob disease. *Proceedings of the National Academy of Sciences USA*, 95, 13239–13241. doi:10.1073/pnas.95.22.13239.

Clavaguera, F., Akatsu, H., Fraser, G., Crowther, R A., Frank, S., Hench, J., . . . and Tolnay, M. (2013). Brain homogenates from human tauopathies induce tau inclusions in mouse brain. *Proceedings of the National Academy of Sciences USA*, Early edition. doi:10.1073/pnas.13-1175110.

Clewley, J. P., Kelly, C. M., Andrews, N., Vogliqi, K., Mallinson, G., Kaisar, M., . . . and Gill, O. N. (2009). Prevalence of disease related prion protein in anonymous tonsil specimens in Britain: cross sectional opportunistic survey. *British Medical Journal*, 338, b1442. doi:10.1136/bmj.b1442.

Colby, D. W., and Prusiner, S. B. (2011). Prions. *Cold Spring Harbor Perspectives in Biology*, 3, a006833. doi:10.1101/cshperspect.a006833.

Collinge, J., Palmer, M. S., and Dryden, A. J. (1991). Genetic predisposition to iatrogenic Creutzfeldt-Jakob disease. *Lancet*, 337, 1441–1442. doi:10.1016/0140-6736(91)93128-V.

Collinge, J., Whitfield, J., McKintosh, E., Beck, J., Mead, S., Thomas, D. J., and Alpers, M. P. (2006). Kuru in the 21st century: an acquired human prion disease with very long incubation periods. *Lancet*, 367, 2068–2074. doi:10.1016/S0140-6736(06)68930-7.

Edgeworth, J. A., Farmer, M., Sicilia, A., Tavares, P., Beck, J., Campbell, T., . . . and Collinge, J. (2011). Detection of prion infection in variant Creutzfeldt-Jakob disease: a blood-based assay. *Lancet*, 377, 487–493. doi:10.1016/S0140- 6736(10)62308-2.

Gajdusek, D. C. (1977). Unconventional viruses and the origin and disappearance of kuru. *Science*, 197, 943–960.

Garruto, R. M., Reiber, C., Alfonso, M. P., Gastrich, H., Needham, K., Sunderman, S., . . . and Shilkret, K. (2008). Risk behaviors in a rural community with a known point-source exposure to chronic wasting disease. *Environmental Health*, 7, 31. doi:10.1186/1476-069X-7-31.

Hilton, D. A., Ghani, A. C., Conyers, L., Edwards, P., McCardle, L., Ritchie, D., . . . and Ironside, J. W. (2004). Prevalence of lymphoreticular prion protein accumulation in UK tissue samples. *Journal of Pathology*, 203, 733–739. doi:10.1002/path.1580.

Hinckley, G. T., Johnson, C. J., Jacobson, K. H., Bartholomay, C., McMahon, K. D., McKenzie, D., . . . and Pedersen, J. A. (2008). Persistence of pathogenic prion protein during simulated wastewater treatment processes. *Environmental Science & Technology*, **42**, 5254–5259. doi:10.1021/es703186e.

Holman, R. C., Belay, E. B., Christensen, K. Y., Maddox, R. A., Minino, A. M., Folkema, A. M., . . . and Schonberger, L. B. (2010). Human prion diseases in the United States. *PLoS ONE*, **5**, e8521. doi:10.1371/journal.pone.0008521.

Ironside, J. W. (2012). Variant Creutzfeldt-Jakob disease: an update. *Folia Neuropathologica*, **50**, 50–56.

Ironside, J. W., Bishop, B. T., Connolly, K., Hegazy, D., Lowrie, S., Le Grice, M., . . . and Hilton, D. A. (2006). Variant Creutzfeldt-Jakob disease: prion protein genotype analysis of positive appendix tissue samples from a retrospective prevalence study. *British Medical Journal*, **332**, 1186–1188. doi:10.1136/bmj.38804.511644.55.

Kariv-Inbal, Z., Ben-Hur, T., Grigoriadis, N. C., Engelstein, R., and Gabizon, R. (2006). Urine from scrapie-infected hamsters comprises low levels of prion infectivity. *Neurodegenerative Diseases*, **3**, 123–128. doi:10.1159/000094770.

Kaski, D., Mead, S.; Hyare, H., Cooper, S., Jampana, R., Overell, J., . . . and Rudge, P. (2009). Variant CJD in an individual heterozygous for PRNP codon 129. *Lancet*, **374**, 2128. doi:10.1016/S0140-6736(09)61568-3.

Kong, Q., Huang, S., Zou, W., Vanegas, D., Wang, M., Wu. D., . . . and Gambetti, P. (2005). Chronic wasting disease of elk: Transmissibility to humans examined by transgenic mouse models. *Journal of Neuroscience*, **25**, 7944–7949. doi:10.1523/JNEUROSCI.2467-05.2005.

Manuelidis, L., Chakrabarty, T., Miyazawa, K., Nduom, A., and Emmerling, K. (2009). The kuru infectious agent is a unique geographic isolate distinct from Creutzfeldt-Jakob disease and scrapie agents. *Proceedings of the National Academy of Sciences USA*, **106**, 13529–13534. doi:10.1073/pnas.0905825106.

MaWhinney, S., Pape. W. J., Forster, J. E., Anderson, C. A., Bosque, P., and Miller, M. W. (2006). Human prion disease and relative risk associated with chronic wasting disease. *Emerging Infectious Diseases*, **12**, 1527–1535. doi:10.3201/eid1210.060019.

Nathanson, N., Wilesmith, J., and Griot, C. (1997). Bovine spongiform encephalopathy (BSE): causes and consequences of a common source epidemic. *American Journal of Epidemiology*, **145**, 959–969.

Palmer, M. S., Dryden, A. J., Hughes, J. T., and Collinge, J. (1991). Homozygous prion protein genotype predisposes to sporadic Creutzfeldt-Jakob disease. *Nature*, **352**, 340–342. doi:10.1038/352340a0.

Pedersen, J. A., and Somerville, R. (2012) Why and how are TSEs sometimes spread via environmental routes? In *Decontamination of prions*. Deslys, J.-P., Pocchiari, M., Reisner, D., and Somerville, R. (eds.), 19–37. Düsseldorf, Germany: Düsseldorf University Press.

Race, B., Meade-White, K. D., Miller, M. W., Barbian, K. D., Rubenstein, R., LaFauci, G., . . . and Chesebro, B. (2009). Susceptibilities of nonhuman primates to chronic wasting disease. *Emerging Infectious Diseases*, **15**, 1366–1376. doi:10.3201/eid1509.090253.

Saá, P., Castilla, J., and Soto C. (2006). Presymptomatic detection of prions in blood. *Science*, **313**, 92–94. doi:10.1126/science.1129051.

Sandberg, M. K., Al-Doujaily, H., Sigurdson, C. J., Glatzel, M., O'Malley, C., Powell, C., . . . and Collinge, J. (2010). *Journal of General Virology*, **91**, 2651–2657. doi:10.1099/vir.0.024380-0.

Sano, K., Satoh, K., Atarashi, R., Takashima, H., Iwasaki, Y., Yoshida, M., . . . and Nishida, N. (2013). Early detection of abnormal prion protein in genetic human prion diseases now possible using real-time QUIC assay. *PLoS ONE*, **8**, e54915. doi:10.1371/journal.pone.0054915.

Schneider, K., Fangerau, H., Michaelsen, B., and Raab, W. H.-M. (2008). The early history of the transmissible spongiform encephalopathies exemplified by scrapie. *Brain Research Bulletin*, **77**, 343–355. doi:10.1016/j.brainresbull.2008.09.012.

Seeger, H., Heikenwalder, M., Zeller, N., Kranich, J., Schwarz, P., . . . and Aguzzi, A. (2005). Coincident scrapie infection and nephritis lead to urinary prion excretion. *Science*, **310**, 324–326. doi:10.1126/science.1118829.

Seidel, B., Thomzig, A., Buschmann, A., Groschup, M. H., Peters, R., Beekes, M., Terytze, K. (2007). Scrapie agent (strain 263K) can transmit disease via the oral route after persistence in soil over years. *PLoS ONE*, **2**, e435. doi:10.1371/journal.pone.0000435.

Soto, C. (2012). Transmissible proteins: Expanding the heresy. *Cell*, **149**, 968–977. doi:10.1016/j.cell.2012.05.007.

Tamgüney, G., Giles, K., Bouzamondo-Bernstein, E., Bosque, P. J., Miller, M. W., Safar, J. G., . . . and Prusiner, S. B. (2006). Transmission of elk and deer prions to transgenic mice. *Journal of Virology*, 80, 9104–9114. doi:10.1128/JVI.00098-06.

Taylor, D. M. (2000). Inactivation of transmissible degenerative encephalopathy agents: a review. *Veterinary Journal*, **159**, 10–17.

Van Dorsselaer, A., Carapito, C., Delalande, F., Schaeffer-Reiss, C. Thierse, D., . . . and Cashman, N. R. (2011). Detection of prion protein in urine-derived injectable fertility products by a targeted proteomic approach. *PLoS ONE*, 6, e17815. doi:10.1371/journal.pone.0017815.

Ward, H. J. T., Everington, D., Cousens, S. N., Smith-Bathgate, B., Leitch, M., Cooper, S., . . . and Will, R. G. (2006). Risk factors for variant Creutzfeldt-Jakob disease: a case-control study. *Annals of Neurology*, 59, 111–120.

Watts, J. C., Balachandran, A., and Westaway, D. (2006). The expanding universe of prion diseases. *PLoS Pathogens*, 2, e26. doi:10.1371/journal.ppat.0020026.

Will, R. G., Ironside, J. W., Zeidler, M., Cousens, S. N., Estibeiro, K., Alperovitch, A., . . . and Smith, P. G. (1996). A new variant of Creutzfeldt-Jakob disease in the UK. *Lancet*, *347*, 921–925.

Wilson, R. Plinston, C., Hunter, N., Casalone, C., Corona, C. Tagliavini, F., . . . and Barron, R. M. (2012). Chronic wasting disease and atypical forms of bovine spongiform encephalopathy and scrapie are not transmissible to mice expressing wild-type levels of human prion protein. *Journal of General Virology*, **93**, 1624–1629. doi:10.1099/vir.0.042507-0.

Xing, Y., Nakamura, A., Chiba, T., Kogishi, K., Matsushita, T., Li, F., . . . and Higuchi, K. (2001). Transmission of mouse senile amyloidosis. *Laboratory Investigation*, **81**, 493–499.

Zhang, B., Une, Y., Fu, X., Yan, J., Ge, F., Yao, J., . . . and Higuchi, K. (2008). Fecal transmission of AA amyloidosis in the cheetah contributes to high incidence of disease. *Proceedings of the National Academy of Sciences USA*, **105**, 7263–7268. doi:10.1073/pnas.0800367105.

Carnivore's Game

Rosalyn W. Berne

Suzie has grown accustomed to hearing the conversations held around her, without participating in them. It's not that she doesn't have anything to say but more that when she does speak up, people don't seem to understand her. Plus, talking has become a bit of a strain. These days she prefers to observe.

On a particularly odd day in May, the weather changes suddenly from unseasonably cool to sweltering. In the course of two hours the temperature rises from 60 degrees to 86 degrees Fahrenheit. Suzie feels it happen. She'd been wearing a sweater because it seemed chilly. Now she feels the hot sun against her skin, and her arms are turning bright red.

As the sun begins to set, a bright, yellow glow pours itself across the tall grasses on the field below. Suzie likes the way the late daylight makes everything glow. She turns her chin upward, noticing the dark branches above her and how they sway ever so gently in the breeze.

"Are you hungry, Suzie?" she hears a voice ask, coming from behind her. She wonders who this Suzie might be and whether this person is indeed hungry. "You're becoming skin and bones, old girl. Now come on in here and get yourself something to eat," the voice continues. Suzie wishes it would stop; it's confusing. She can't fathom what skin and bones this woman means. Is someone cooking up a pot of meat? There's been no hunting since last season. And the farm animals out in the fields aren't looking too appetizing these days.

Suzie feels a tapping on her shoulder, and it irritates her. She pushes the hand away and grunts. Another voice comes up to her side, the lips placed close to her cheek. "Mwah," she hears. *This must be Ben. He's a good boy . . . always has been. Ever since his Papa got waylaid it's been extra helpful to have him around.*

"Why is she bothering me this way?" Suzie asks her son about the woman who is still talking nonsense—"she" being Suzie's sister Emma, who had come all the way across the state to visit, having been warned of Suzie's rapidly declining condition. It was frightening—just like with Suzie's husband, who passed away so quickly that there was hardly time to get used to the idea of him being gone, especially not for Suzie. Ever since that Saturday last month when they put Papa in the ground, she spends most of every day on the porch in anticipation of his truck coming out from behind the barn and pulling up in front of the house.

"Emma, they don't know what to make of it," Ben shares. "They even did a genetic scan. Nothing. There's no explaining it."

"They did a what?" Emma replies, stroking her sister's long, red hair.

This woman seems worried about something.

"Chip technology. You know, studying individual DNA to find genetic mutations," Ben explains.

She must be nervous, the way she holds her hand so stiff combing my hair with her fingers like this. Suzie pushes Emma's arm away from her then begins to stroke her hair herself.

"Looks like Alzheimer's disease to me," Emma replies as she steps away from her sister, leaning her back against the peeling white paint on the clapboard wall of the house. "Except that she's too young for that, isn't she?"

"Too young, and also born too late. That got cured years ago with a plant-based synthetic compound. First it was tested on living neurons. Then they figured out that it could treat Alzheimer's disease."

"Now don't go getting all technical on me," Emma chides her nephew.

"Looks to me more like what made Papa sick," he replies.

"Oh!" Suzie adds, her attention more on the tangles between her fingers than on what Ben was saying. "Papa on his way home?"

It dawns on her now who that person is. Suzie recognizes her estranged sister. She never liked her too much. *What is she doing here?*

"I came out to let you know that the steaks are on," Ben says. "They should be ready by now."

"Good. I'm about starved," Emma replies.

"Let's get her back into the house," Ben suggests. "Maybe the smell of food will stimulate her hunger."

It's been so quiet in the house lately, feeling so strange and empty. I'd rather stay out here and wait for Papa to come back.

"She always liked a good cut of meat," Emma says, passing her hand over her sister's shoulder. "Back when we were little girls our daddy would smoke it. Your mother would clean the meat from a bone 'til there wasn't a bit of flesh left on it." Ben chuckled.

"Maybe that's why she married my father," he said rubbing his chin.

"What are you talking about, Ben?"

"Well, Papa liked to hunt. He preferred to kill what he ate, on principle. He always said you don't know that what you are eating was once a living animal when you buy it all pretty in a plastic wrap from the store. Mama thought that was an indication of his virtue."

"I suppose," Emma replied. "But your mother was always overly moralistic."

Ben ignored the comment and continued. "He'd take his fresh game straight to the shed and dress it, you know, getting out the vital organs. He tried to teach me, but I didn't have the stomach for it. But I watched him skin it and then hang it to cool and firm up. Papa said we'd have to wait until it cured because that is what makes it tender. Eventually he'd retrieve it and put it in his barbecue pit. Then he and Mama would play their game."

"Which reminds me," Emma interrupts, "the sauce you've prepared smells great."

"Hope it tastes as good as it smells," Ben returns.

"So what was the game?" Emma asks.

Ben's smile softens, and his lips pull taut. A frown forms of his brows. "'The Game- game' is what they called it."

"What?" Emma asked as she tried through gestures to coax her sister up from the rocking chair. "Come on now, Suzie. Let's go inside and eat."

"Papa would bring his barbecue to the table. He'd tell Mama to taste it before asking any questions. After her first bite he'd say, 'You liked it didn't you!' And Mama would invariably grin, licking her lips in an exaggerated way to indicate yes. Then Papa would challenge her by saying, 'Now guess what kind of game it is!' She only sometimes got it right: wild turkey, possum, quail, venison, duck, fox, bear, or groundhog. Once in a while she'd surprise him, like when she correctly guessed cougar. But the time Mama guessed rabbit and it turned out to be squirrel, Mama cried. She said squirrels weren't for eating and that they didn't cause anyone any trouble, just minding their business, collecting and burying nuts. Papa told her, 'Anything that can run is game for my gun.' She never again played his game."

"Let's get that steak on a plate in front of her," Emma suggested. "I think once she takes a bite she'll know how famished she is."

What in the world might she be talking about, and why did this strange woman just pat me on the head? "Ben! Do something about that horse that keeps climbing up on this porch," Suzie yells out, suddenly standing from her rocker. "Go on, git! NOW!" she screeches as if frightened, or in distress, "If you don't get away right now, Papa's gonna come back and prepare you for eatin'!" Neither Ben nor Emma responds.

"Did you understand what your mother said?" Emma asks Ben. "I couldn't quite make out her words."

"Something about wanting to ride a horse, I think," Ben returns. "Now you see for yourself what it's been like with her for the past few days. And why I thought you'd better come. I can hardly make out what's she's saying half the time, especially when she gets upset or excited."

Suzie stands pounding her foot hard against the porch floorboards, waving her arms wildly in all directions. "He's coming closer. What does he want? That horse is too heavy to be up here on this porch. He'll destroy it. Get him off, Ben. Get him off now!"

"It's okay, Mama," Ben says as he heads in her direction. He takes her arm, though unsteadily. "It's getting dark out now," he speaks gently, placing a kiss on his mother's head. "Ben, you are staggering!" Emma exclaims.

Chapter 5

Climate Change and the Future of Freshwater

David L. Feldman
Department of Planning, Policy and Design, School of Social Ecology,
300G Social Ecology I, University of California, Irvine,
CA 92697-7075, USA
feldmand@uci.edu

While climate change may not seem to be a direct focus of biotechnology, its impact on surface water, drinking water, and groundwater quality is already becoming of significance to the field. Changes in temperature and precipitation patterns have an adverse effect on water quality, with higher air temperatures, earlier snowmelt, and decreases in precipitation contributing to widespread drought and an increase in the frequency of floods. If sea levels continue to rise, the salinity of coastal rivers and bays will also increase, causing saltwater intrusion into fresh groundwater resources. Biotechnology uses a broad array of tools that are applied to a wide spectrum of purposes, including health care and pharmaceuticals, food production, and other agriculture. Biotechnology can also play a role in addressing the water quality and water scarcity issues that could arise

Creating Life from Life: Biotechnology and Science Fiction
Edited by Rosalyn W. Berne
Copyright © 2015 Pan Stanford Publishing Pte. Ltd.
ISBN 978-981-4463-58-4 (Hardcover), 978-981-4463-59-1 (eBook)
www.panstanford.com

with global climate change, such as with drought-resistant plants, pathogen detection, bioremediation and biotreatment of wastewater, surface and coastal waters, and aquifers. David Feldman takes a step back from the particulars of the possible scientific solutions to consider freshwater from the broader perspective of adaptation.

Imagine that in the not-too-distant future familiar patterns of rain and snow dramatically shift due to human activities that generate greenhouse gases. Carbon dioxide and methane emissions would alter the climate in various ways: Global average temperatures would rise, for example, and dramatic changes in precipitation could adversely affect the world's freshwater supply. Rainfall intensity could increase in some regions and decline in others, while the seasonal balance between snow and rain might also shift, affecting local economies. Higher temperatures could increase evaporation and transpiration (the rate at which plants "give up" moisture to the surrounding air). Both would result in less soil moisture, affecting farming and ranching.

Over longer time periods, shifts in the vegetation cover over entire regions—from forests to grasslands or even grasslands to deserts—might occur. Accelerated melting of polar and glacial ice—another probable result of climate change—would lead to greater sea-level rise and more saltwater intrusion into coastal estuaries, affecting fisheries and threatening the quality of urban drinking water supplies (Climate Institute, 2010).

Many scientists believe these changes are not only likely scenarios but that current protracted drought in some regions and unprecedented flooding in others are harbingers of worse to come. While the debate over whether, and to what extent, any given climatic event may be attributable to global climate change is far from settled, there is a growing consensus that the increasing frequency of water-related extreme climate events is probably the result of human-induced climate change. As one scientist pointed out, the problem is comparable to "asking whether steroids helped a baseball player hit a home run at the bottom of the ninth inning of the World Series." If the player were able to hit home runs before taking steroids, it would be impossible to know whether any particular home run could be traced directly to performance-enhancing drugs. However, at the end of the season, it would be clear that the player hit home runs more often. "That's what we have here . . . we've juiced the world's climate system by putting these gases in the atmosphere" (Morin, 2012).

Worsening conditions for the world's freshwater due to climate change demand concerted, imaginative, science-based solutions—particularly in poorer, less developed countries. This essay examines prospects for adapting to these changes and our ability to survive them. It also examines how translation of climate knowledge is helping spur adaptation efforts at various spatial levels. These experiences point to the challenges in adaptation *and* the further adversity we face if we don't.

What Is Adaptation?

Adaptation is the pursuit of measures to enhance our ability to manage the water supply and attenuate demands in the face of climate uncertainty. It requires imaginative management as well as good science, and it depends on the ability to translate knowledge into common language useful to decision makers and the public. Moreover, it may embrace activities undertaken for reasons other than climate change.

Adaptation can take place anywhere. As regard climate and water, we'll focus on two venues where climate variability is already affecting freshwater management, megacities and large river basins experiencing drought and/or flooding.

Megacities and Freshwater

Megacities are urban centers composed of tens of millions of people. A growing phenomenon in developing nations, especially, where some 80% of the planet's urban population resides—the urban populace of Africa, Asia, and Latin America alone has swelled fivefold since 1950 (Satterthwaite, 2000; United Nations Population Fund, 2007). Large cities generally, and megacities in particular, are often located some distance from the water sources they need. As a result they often divert water from outlying rural areas, which in turn often produce the food and fiber that directly supports these teeming populations.

In recent years, many cities in developing and developed countries have begun taking measures to secure more resilient water supplies. While partly driven by climate change concerns, the immediate drivers of these adaptation efforts are population growth, the need to share available supplies with neighboring communities, and political pressure to restore threatened habitat. While many examples could be cited, four large cities— representing an array of baseline climates—typify some of these pressures: New York, Tokyo, Los Angeles, and Mexico City.

Since the 1980s, New York—a "wet" city (an average of 50 inches of precipitation per year, half of that in the form of snow)— has found that even relative abundance can become a deficit, given the population growth and antiquated infrastructure. Since the late 1970s the city has undertaken measures to reduce residential water use (which has declined by 30% in 35 years), repair aqueducts reaching the Catskills and Croton watersheds to forestall leaks, and evaluate possible impacts of climate change. Working with local universities and environmental organizations, officials are trying to determine how sea-level rise and storm surges will affect water and wastewater infrastructure, how higher temperatures and lower precipitation will affect public supply as well as ecosystem health, and whether capital planning needs to adapt to these changes can be anticipated (New York City Department of Environmental Protection, 2010, 1998; New York State Department of Environmental Conservation, 2010a, 2010b; Shultz, 2007).

Tokyo—one of the world's largest cities—is also located in a traditionally wet climate, receiving some 60 inches of precipitation per year, most of which falls as rain during midsummer. Since World War II, rapid in-migration and economic growth dramatically increased water demands; at the same time planners were led to pave over and cover small waterways to facilitate urban expansion. Increased consumption has led to a decline in groundwater and land subsidence. Since the 1980s, concerns over climate change—including local "heat island" effects from urbanization, leading to additional energy use—have prompted the introduction of large-scale wastewater reuse, storm-water harvesting for nonpotable needs, restrictions on groundwater withdrawals, and more aggressive water conservation (Bureau of Waterworks, Tokyo Metropolitan Government, 2012; Blanco, McCarney, Parnell, Schmidt, and Seto, 2011).

By comparison, Los Angeles and Mexico City, located in historically dryer climates, are facing comparable, if graver, challenges. Receiving some 15 inches of rain per year, utilities in the Los Angeles basin have long employed public education and outreach programs to reduce residential water use. In 2011, average daily demands remained the same as in 1980, despite 1.1 million more people living in Los Angeles County. Storm-water capture and wastewater reuse are among additional alternatives being explored, and climate change is now embraced in regional planning efforts such as those by the Metropolitan Water District of Southern California, the area's principal water provider since the 1930s. How climate change will complicate water rights exchanges with outlying rural areas and affect water rights acquired from regional agricultural users is being explored. How seismic events might disrupt already precarious imported supplies is also being examined (Los Angeles Department of Water and Power, 2009, 2010a, 2010b).

Finally, Mexico City, one of the world's largest cities (>20 million) and recipient of some 28 inches of rainfall annually, exemplifies the complexities of adaptation in Third World cities. Plans long underway to adapt to growing water demands are now being adjusted for climate change. Unsurprisingly, most of these plans hinge on additional water transfers from outlying regions to recharge local aquifers and surface reservoirs. Efforts are also being pursued to reduce residential water demand, use more reclaimed wastewater for local agriculture and nonpotable uses, and employ storm-water capture for groundwater recharge and near immediate local uses. How effective these measures will prove to be is subject to considerable debate (Downs, Mazari-Hiriart, Dominguez-Mora, and Suffet, 2000; Tortajada and Casteian, 2003; Institut de Recherche pour la Developpement, 2012).

River Basins and Adaptation

Two ambitious examples of extensive basin-wide adaptation efforts to manage drought and flooding—partly induced by climate change—are found in Nigeria and Bangladesh. In 2002, the World Conservation Union and the U.K.'s foreign assistance agency partnered with the government of Nigeria in an effort focused on the Hadejia-Jama'are basin to build "local water resources management capacity" in a region long suffering alternation of flooding and drought. Among the unique features of this Joint Wetlands Livelihood project are improving use of local knowledge; demonstrating pilot-scale, best-management practices to restore the region's economy and ecology by showing how to conduct dry-season grazing, recharge groundwater, and restore waterfowl habitat. Most innovatively, local-level forums comprising farmers, women's groups, and villagers engage in community-level training, apply local knowledge to water management, and directly participate in policy making by role-playing scenarios to manage parts of the watershed in ways that maximize equity while protecting agricultural productivity (Muhammad, Yahaya, Yahya, and Abba, n.d.; Lankford, 2005).

By contrast, the Bengali Delta of Bangladesh consistently suffers from too much water, with chronic flooding from cyclones and monsoonal storms a too-frequent occurrence. While thousands have died from floods, there is fear that sea-level rise caused by melting glaciers will worsen floods and displace upward of 15% of the country's 160 million. Because the Ganges and Brahmaputra deltas constantly shift, securing their banks and protecting rich farmland is difficult. In the 1990s, a World Bank plan backed by France, Japan, and the U.S., proposed some 8,000 km of dikes to control these streams at an estimated cost of $10 billion, together with sea walls to resist cyclone-induced waves. Local farmers opposed these plans because their lands would be taken, while the Intergovernmental Panel on Climate Change criticized them because local soils were too unstable to support such efforts.

As an alternative, local villagers and farmers, working with NGOs, including U.K.-based Practical Action and U.S.-based CARE, advanced local-scale programs to adapt to flooding, including 2-foot-high concrete plinths topped with inexpensive jute panel–walled homes that are less likely to be washed away by tropical storms, reintroduction of formerly forgotten farming techniques such as baira cultivation and floating gardens suited to areas subject to lengthy inundation, introduction of salt-tolerant varieties of rice, and conversion of some paddies to shrimp and crab raising. These innovations would not have been introduced without incorporating the knowledge of local farmers and villagers.

Translating Climate Science

Translating climate knowledge to make it useful to lay audiences is a huge adaptation challenge. There's a huge gap in the way scientists talk about climate change and the way farmers, villagers, urban residents, and other lay audiences talk about water problems. Translation is an effort to literally simplify science. Efforts taking place in Brazil and the Nile basin in Africa show how this may be done effectively. Since the 1990s, the northeast Brazilian state of Ceara has sought to institute legal reforms in response to drought and competing water claims—

and to foster collaboration between scientists and local farmers. In coordination with federal agencies, a series of participatory management councils have been introduced in the lower Jaguaribe-Banabmuiú River basin to negotiate water allocation agreements among users.

In a departure from traditional top-down decision making, *técnicos* (staff scientists) work with farmers to combine local knowledge of drought/flood impacts with long-term expert weather predictions and help farmers and local governments better manage reservoirs, flood, and drought. Results have thus far yielded a willingness among farmers to share management of local water supplies, while the state water management authority permits locals to monitor conditions. Local users, for their part, hold greater trust in state-level information (Lemos and Oliveira, 2004, 2005).

Since 1998, the 10 countries of Africa's Nile basin (Kenya, Burundi, Rwanda, Tanzania, Eritrea, Ethiopia, Sudan, Egypt, Uganda, and Congo) have tried to negotiate an agreement to share the waters of the basin equitably, acknowledging the needs of fast-growing upstream countries, while respecting— where possible—the established rights of Sudan and Egypt. The latter—which have the basin's largest populations—are reluctant to relinquish withdrawal rights, while upstream Ethiopia is committed to harnessing tributaries for hydroelectricity and water supply without Egypt's permission, creating additional friction. While solutions are debated, Lake Victoria, a major source of the Nile, falls some 2.5 m every 3 years due to climate change.

Despite such acrimony, some adaptation is occurring in *sub-basins*, including international support for irrigation improvements, groundwater management, and rural electrification projects. Moreover, local communities, NGOs, scientists, and aid organizations are working together to design solutions, identify funding sources, and share information (*Nile Basin Initiative*, 2010; Alive2green, 2009; Fleishman and Linthicum, 2010).

Conclusions

Prospects for climate change are compelling communities across the globe to adapt to freshwater shortages and other alterations. Cities and river basins are actually well suited for undertaking adaptation efforts if the political will can be found to mobilize hard choices. Adaptation will require 1) better communication between scientists and end users, facilitated by efforts to formalize dialogue between them (e.g., Brazil, Nigeria); 2) adaptive management—an approach emphasizing social learning and incremental solutions that are reversible if they fail (e.g., Bangladesh, Nile basin, megacities); and 3) recognition that sound knowledge and effective collaboration go together (Robinson, 2007; Belt, 2011)—experts must reach out to local water users and embrace cultural, social, and ethical concerns if the world is to face global climate change's impacts on freshwater.

References

Alive2green (2009). The rights to the river. *The Sustainable Water Resources e-journal*, **1**(2), www.waterresource.co.za/index.php?option=com_Content.

Belt, D. (2011). The coming storm. *National Geographic*, **219**(5), 58–83.

Blanco, H., McCarney, P., Parnell, S., Schmidt, M., and Seto, K. C. (2011). The role of urban land in climate change. *Climate Change and Cities: First Assessment Report of the Urban Climate Change Research Network*, 240.

Bureau of Waterworks, Tokyo Metropolitan Government (2012). *Water Supply in Tokyo*, http://www.waterworks.metro.tokyo.jp/eng/supply/index.html.

Climate Institute (2010). *Water*, http://www.climate.org/topics/water.html.

Downs, T. M., Mazari-Hiriart, M., Dominguez-Mora, R., and Suffet, H. (2000). Sustainability of least cost policies for meeting Mexico City's future water demand. *Water Resources Research*, **36**(8), 2321–2339.

Fleishman, J., and Linthicum, K. (2010, September 12). Demands on the Nile imperil Egypt's lifeline. *Los Angeles Times*, A-1, 6–7.

Institut de Recherche pour la Developpement (2012). *Water Supplies to Mexico City,* http://en.ird.fr/the-research/the-research-projects/water-supplies-to-mexico-city.

Lankford, B. (2005). *Facilitation of Water Sharing Arrangements in the Hadejia Jama'are Komadugu Yobe Basin (HJKYB): With the River Basin Game Dialogue Tool.* Final report. Norwich, U.K.: Overseas Development Group (ODG), School of Development Studies, University of East Anglia.

Lemos M. C., and Oliveira, J. L. F. (2004). Can water reform survive politics? Institutional change and river basin management in Ceará, Northeast Brazil. *World Development*, 32(12), 2121–2137.

Lemos, M. C., and Oliveira, J. L. F. (2005). Water reform across the state/society divide: the case of Ceará, Brazil. *International Journal of Water Resources Development*, 21(1), 93–107.

Los Angeles Department of Water and Power (2009). *Mandatory Water Conservation: Fact Sheet,* May 4.

Los Angeles Department of Water and Power (2010a). *Urban Water Management Plan,* www.ladwp.com.

Los Angeles Department of Water and Power (2010b). *The Story of the Los Angeles Aqueduct*, http://wsoweb.ladwp.com/Aqueduct/historyoflaa/.

Morin, M. (2012, October 12). Some climate scientists, in a shift, link weather to global warming. *Los Angeles Times*, http://articles.latimes.com/2012/oct/12/science/la-sci-weather-climate-change-20121013.

Muhammad, J. C., Yahaya, D. K., Yahya, B. K., and Abba, J. G. (n.d.). *Water Management Issues in the Hadejia-Jama'are-Komadugu-Yobe Basin: DFID-JWL and Stakeholders Experience in Information Sharing, Reaching Consensus and Physical Interventions*, http://www.iwmi.cgiar.org/research_impacts/Research_Themes/BasinWaterManagement/RIPARWIN/PDFs/14%20Muhammad%20Chiroma%20SS%20FINAL%20EDIT.pdf.

New York City Department of Environmental Protection (1998). *Drought Management Plan and Rules,* December.

New York City Department of Environmental Protection (2010). *New York City 2010 Drinking Water Supply and Quality Report*. Flushing, NY: Author, http://www.nyc.gov/html/dep/pdf/wsstate10.pdf.

New York State Department of Environmental Conservation (2010a). *New York City Watershed Program*, http://www.dec.ny.gov/land58597.htm.

New York State Department of Environmental Conservation (2010b). *Facts about the New York City Watershed*, http://www.dec.ny.gov/lands/58524.html.

Nile Basin Initiative (2010), http://www.nilebasin.org.

Robinson, S. (2007, November 19). How Bangladesh survived a flood. *New York Times*, http://www.time.com/time/world/article/0,8599,1685330,00.html#ixzz1ctqiWiPs.

Satterthwaite, D. (2000). Will most people live in cities? *British Medical Journal*, **321**(7269), 1143–1145, http://www.pubmedcentral.nih.gov/articlerender.fcgi?artid+1118907.

Shultz, H. (2007). *Some Facts on the New York City Water and Sewer Supply System*. New York, NY: Citizens' Housing and Planning Council.

Tortajada, C., and Casteian, E. (2003). Water management for a megacity: Mexico City metropolitan area. *Ambio*, **32**(2), 124–129.

United Nations Population Fund (2007). *State of World Population 2007: Unleashing the Potential of Urban Growth*. NY: Author.

Negotiations

Rosalyn W. Berne

IT WAS THE KIND of heat that felt dangerous. Ashley sat still, engulfed by its intensity, as she waited for her host to arrive. The rainy season had not yet begun in Lagos, although it was already late May.

"In fact," said the man sitting next to her in the aisle seat of the transatlantic shuttle, "we haven't had monsoon rains in over two years."

Ashley was interested to hear that. She was deeply concerned. It was her job to understand the situation and to offer possible solutions. She knew the technical aspects well, but hearing a personal perspective would provide deeper insight.

"Oh really?" she replied. The man nodded and continued.

"There's been no regular rainfall since they starting relocating clouds from the coast to where the government officials live in Abuja. Conditions got worse when they moved more clouds to the agricultural regions."

"No surprise about that," Ashley replied.

"Yes, to ensure irrigation of the cocoa plant, one of our most precious commodities," he continued. "Cocoa farmers can no longer depend upon the rain. And as for the city residents, water flow is low because the rivers that supply our water have not kept up with the demand."

"With no rain and no clouds, and falling dam levels, what do you do for drinking water?" Ashley asked, feeling increasingly anxious. Her purpose in making this trip was to offer her engineering expertise. This is what she'd trained for. But most of all, she wanted to help ease the suffering of the people. The man loosened his colorful tie.

"Treated municipal water is available for a price," he explained. "I am truly blessed."

Ashley gnawed on a split fingernail. "I think there are other explanations for why you have water and others don't," she returned.

The man picked up a spoon and stirred sugar and cream into the cup of hot tea before him, commenting that tea drinking in Nigeria is a tradition left by the British. He took three sips, slurping the warm liquid as if to signal his enjoyment. Putting the cup back down, he continued.

"My friend, life in the coastal city has become very difficult. Those of us who can afford the water are resented by those who can't. Sometimes we have even been threatened with violence. Every day, more people arrive from the north, requesting water, but they have no funds to buy it."

"Do you personally have the water you need?" Ashley clarified.

"I do, usually, yes, and the same is with others who can handle the tariff. The ones who can't have no choice but to wait for the rains."

"May I ask how much the water costs you?"

"In naira or in dollars?" the man asked.

"Dollars would be helpful."

The man looked away for a moment and cleared his throat before speaking again. Lowering his voice, he spoke slowly. Ashley was enchanted by the melodic sound of his distinctive accent.

"What we refer to as 'low-grade water' runs from 2 dollars and 50 cents to 6 dollars and 50 cents per liter, depending on the rains. That's the rate for high-density urban dwellers. The Water Authority provides their water by pipeline. The standard grade is for bathing, hair washing, and laundry. Recycled gray water is used for toilets."

"Does everyone in Lagos have access to the authority's water?" Ashley knew the answer because she'd been prepared for her visit by the West African team at the home office. But she wondered how an ordinary Nigerian citizen might respond to such a question.

"Not everyone," he returned. "The pipes go to high-rise residential buildings, most single-family homes, and businesses. Those in the water villages live in houseboats, and they have plumbing for running water. And others, who live in communities outside the reach of the water mains, have to rely on what their cisterns can hold. Their owners pay an annual tax of 500 dollars for the right to collect rainwater."

"What?" Ashley burst out in a shout. Embarrassed, she quickly calmed herself. Somehow her team had missed this fact. "Since when did rain become a government-allocated commodity?" she demanded.

"Since it ceased to fall readily from the sky and was no longer seen as plentiful, that's when, my friend." Ashley shifted her position as much as possible in the narrow coach seat.

"And what about the water you drink and cook with?" she continued.

"For cooking food or making coffee and tea, standard-grade water can be used because it is boiled before use."

"Then what do you pay for water you don't boil, that you drink and put directly into your mouth?" The man peered over the rim of his glasses.

"Why would we drink water without boiling it?" he returned.

"Boiling water takes energy!" she burst out.

"We have plenty of that," he returned. "You must know of our oil."

"Forgive me, sir. Of course I do. Let me explain. Water resources engineering is my line of work. Ideally you should be able to the drink water straight from your tap."

"You say you are an engineer?" he chuckled as he continued. "For brushing teeth we use standard-grade, boiled water. Those who can afford it, and have access to the pipeline, can get a designated tap put into their homes, which provides biotreated, or what we call 'premium,' water. The cost runs between 55 and 68 dollars per liter, depending on the rains and whether the source is the rivers to the north or the sky."

Ashley noted how matter-of-factly he spoke, as if describing the time the mail is delivered or the availability of cloth for his tailored pants, rather than a circumstance of such despair. What she heard was increasingly frustrating. His nonchalance was infuriating. *What happens to the poor while you privileged guzzle down that liquid gold? What makes you entitled to such blessings but not them?*

Ashley wondered about the two-thirds of the population that lived in the city's slums. How did they get along without the rains, especially the children, the invalid, and the elderly? And when the rains did arrive, how could they possibly afford the rainwater tariff?

"I am on my way to Nigeria to help," Ashley offered after a moment's silence. "I am a consultant with an international firm that provides expertise to the water-stressed regions of the world."

"Well done," the man replied, adding a word from his mother tongue. "Dalu."

"Dalu?"

"It means 'thank you' in Igbo. I thank you in advance for what you will try to do."

"I will meet a fellow expert, a Nigerian woman named Nkasi."

"Achibgu?"

"Yes, that's her," Ashley confirmed. "She works for our client in Nigeria."

"I know her," the man returned with a nod. "She is well known for her efforts in the water negotiations. Say my hello to her."

"OK, I will," Ashley replied.

The two did not speak again during the remainder of the flight. Ashley used the time instead to contemplate the challenges ahead of her.

Getting through immigrations was simple enough once Ashley handed three hundred dollars in cash to the official. She'd been told that offering to pay the "fee" would expedite her entry as a first-time visitor. She claimed her bag from the carousel, passed through customs, and then stepped from the conditioned air out into the raw, blazing sun. She quivered from the shock to her senses. *I am here. I am in Africa!* This was her first visit to the continent. Most of her water consultations thus far had been near home, in the southwest region of the U.S. It was hot there, too, but nothing like this heat-on-top-of-heat that was thickened by intense humidity.

She wondered where and when Nkasi would meet her. They had given each other access to their *telepathoughts*, to send and receive messages through the neurowiring buried underneath their skulls, so that they could communicate easily during the flight.

I am running late due to traffic, but I am on my way, Nkasi thought. *Look for the "bumble-bee." That's what I call my footwagon.*

OK. I will wait out front, Ashley thought in response, curious about the meaning of the word "footwagon."

Ashley took a seat on a bench outside the Murtala Muhammed International Airport and waited for her host, Nkasi, to arrive. *It's perfect that there is so much humidity. Exactly what I am counting on,* she thought, clutching the bag that carried the novel device.

Nearly an hour passed. The sun bore down ruthlessly, the rays penetrating her vulnerable skin. Ashley sat totally still, as if doing so would keep her cooler. Despite the white cotton sleeves of her shirt, the broad white hat on her head, and the sunscreen protection she rubbed on her arms, legs, face, chest, and neck, Ashley's flesh was burning.

Nkasi sent a thought that she had moved only a few miles in her car and still was over half a mile away. Ashley thought about going back inside the terminal, and Nkasi let her know that it was best she wait; she would be there soon. Ashley decided to remain where she was.

Her throat parched, Ashley reached into her bag for the water she purchased during the trip. "Damn it," she mumbled under her breath, noting how little was left. She leaned her head back and tapped the last few drops onto her tongue before tossing the empty container into a nearby bin.

"Madam, please, water for you," said a man walking toward her. "For you, madam, only 1000 Naira. A cool, refreshing sachet of premium water."

She noticed the vender's curly hair, his pointed nose, and his thin lips. *Fulani, the once nomadic people who conquered the Hausa in the north and brought Islam to Nigeria . . .* She noticed his skin, blackened by genetic adaptation. To stay safe, stay dark; his DNA knew what to do. His head was wrapped in green and black woven fabric. *What is he doing in Lagos?* She remembered what the team told her about the recent migrations and the 10-year drought that persisted in the north.

He held a sachet out in front of her, a clear plastic bag filled with about 6 ounces of water. She was tempted to take it but instead scoffed.

"Get away from here," Ashley scolded him. She would not let this shyster take advantage of her.

"Not to worry, it's purified," the vendor assured her. His eyes appeared sincere. But how could she be certain of its quality? "For you, madam, only 1000 naira," he repeated.

"Are you kidding me?" Ashley replied. "Why would I pay over 6 US dollars for barely a few gulps of water?"

"Madam, it's a very good price, end-of-the-day discount. Regular price 1500 naira. Please, take the water and drink. It's hot out here under the sun. And you have been sitting for a very long time."

Ashley turned her attention to the traffic as it moved in and out of the airport, and tried to ignore the man in front of her. When the small yellow car with three black stripes on its hood approached, she took hold of her suitcase and jumped up, waving. The smiling woman behind the wheel waved in return, and Ashley felt both welcomed and relieved.

Nkasi pulled up and got out of the car. "I can tell it's you because you are so beautiful," Nkasi declared, opening her arms for a wide embrace. "Welcome to my country!"

Or maybe you can tell it's me because I am the only fair-skinned person around. Ashley thought, and then realized with dismay that she had forgotten to turn off her *telepathought* connection.

"No, no! That's not the reason why," Nkasi replied, laughing. "You look just like the image you project when we talk on the global network." Ashley was ashamed that she felt conspicuous; she had seen no other white people since stepping onto the plane.

As they drove through the city, the two new acquaintances chatted idly, with Nkasi doing most of the talking. They passed a golf club, a country club, lagoons, and sprawling slums before entering onto the Third Mainland Bridge. Exhausted from the seven-hour flight from New York to Lagos, Ashley felt dazed, though excited. But seeing so many uniformed, armed soldiers gave her pause. "Why so much military presence?" she asked.

"Did the home office not inform you?" Nkasi replied. "About the state of emergency we entered yesterday?"

"No, they didn't," Ashley returned. She wondered what this may mean for her visit.

"I honestly wondered why you would still come," Nkasi admitted. "I am so grateful that you are here. The situation is horrible."

"How so?" Ashley asked, wondering if she'd made a mistake in thinking she could make a difference in this desperate situation.

"Ethnic lines are being drawn, and threats of violence increase every day," Nkasi sighed. Releasing one hand from the steering wheel, she rubbed her neck. "I am sure you know of Lake Chad," she continued, "in the northern part of Nigeria. It once spanned over 520 square miles, but now it is barely a puddle. And do you know about the industrial southwest? Where they do the oil drilling? Those people who live there have nothing to drink. They are dying every day by the thousands."

"Maybe what I have can help them, too."

"Ashley, it's too late for that. They are living under Nigeria's version of Marshal Law. And we will NOT be visiting there."

"But everywhere I look I see water. It seems Lagos is surrounded by water!" Ashley returned. "You could supply your whole country from this resource."

"People always assume that. But the waters you see in the lagoons and the ocean are not fit for human consumption," Nkasi explained. "We built a few nuclear desalination plants, for low-grade water use, but the tremors made running them too dangerous."

"The problem is much more severe than I realized," Ashley mumbled.

Nkasi turned onto a secondary street. "I will try to avoid some traffic," she explained. Even the road chosen as a detour was dense with traffic. Ashley rolled up her window. The air was very dusty. The sound was overwhelming, as if every driver was pounding on his or her horn. Men and women walked on the sides of the road, with their babies wrapped in cloth and strapped to their backs. Men and women were sleeping on the street.

"What's worse is that because of losing Lake Chad, 50 million people, maybe more, were displaced. Many of them tried to get here but either gave up or died on the way."

"Nkasi, there are other sources of water. Why aren't those being pursued?" Ashley inquired. Nkasi turned her gaze from the traffic outside to the colleague sitting in the seat to her right.

"Because underground water overdrafts throughout the country left thousands of dysfunctional wells and depleted aquifers. Then came an urgent push by the government to build dams."

"Which led to massive flooding, right?"

"Exactly," Nkasi said. "The wars were inevitable. Masses of people moved here, to the coast, in search of available water."

"I see why they would come here. It appears that you are water wealthy."

Nkasi turned her attention back to the road, saying, "And now you understand that we are not. Our project is my last hope for this crisis."

Ashley grabbed tightly her bag on her lap, saying, "Oh yes, we can put our hope in this."

Ashley shared about how the situation in the southwest U.S. was also getting serious, with anger and desperation increasing daily. And of how the box would be needed at home, too. The two discussed recent events and things of interest to most professional young women like themselves: earning enough money to live on comfortably, finding a place to call home at a safe distance from the water skirmishes, and, hopefully, finding someone to share that home with. Having children was not mentioned, as it'd become a taboo subject. Many of those who could do so were choosing not to get pregnant, especially where water was expensive.

"What's that over there?" Ashley asked as they moved past a huge expanse of floating debris, glass, and mud.

"Oh, that's what remains of Victoria Island," Nkasi explained. "It was once restaurants, shopping malls, hotels, bars, banks, night clubs, movie theatres, schools, and luxury apartment buildings. Lots of businesses, lots of millionaires." Tangled wires hung from the tilted rooftops of what had once been high-rise buildings.

"Good gracious," Ashley said, at a loss for anything else to say. "I knew about Victoria Island, but I didn't know it was this bad."

"How could you not? It's our great tragedy. It seems you have come here in relative ignorance, my friend." Nkasi squinted her eyes and pursed her lips, adding, "Many thousands died."

"I am so sorry. What happened?"

"Heavy downpours and high winds for days and days and days . . . much worse than our usual monsoons. The flooding was sudden, but we anticipated that. But then, after the floodwaters receded came the tremors. They were so strong, shaking the city for three days straight. Then came the collapsing land, spontaneous sinkholes everywhere, and finally buildings began to topple and sink. Our geologists never expected that. Many of the survivors left Lagos all together and returned to their villages in the East and West. Ikoyi Island was destroyed, too," she explained, pointing in the direction it used to be.

"Those who could afford to relocated to the Banana Island," she continued, "which sustained much less damage."

"Banana Island . . . ooh, tropical sounding. Was it a pretty fancy place?"

"Another land reclamation project. And yes, it was very fancy, as you say. Only for the very rich and powerful."

Ashley, rolling the car window down again, was struck by the scent of electricity, as if the air itself was charged.

The trees lining the streets of Weibo Road stood motionless. Strokes of green formed a backdrop against the concrete structures, representatives of a life form that adapted to withstand the drought. "Welcome to my home," Nkasi offered as they arrived at the pink and turquoise concrete house. Nkasi had found an oasis—a two-bedroom home nestled among a crowded megalopolis of high rises. She had found a way of living well, it seemed, in a city of 28 million people. A houseboy, as Nkasi called him, appeared and took Ashley's bag to the guest room and then disappeared from view.

She and Ashley had work to do and not much time to get ready. Hearings were in progress. Riots were threatened. The ministry was advocating water rights for those who had no direct access, but only with a levy of tariffs. People were enraged. Nkasi served Ashley a meal of coconut rice with fish, fresh mango, stewed vegetables, and red beans. She debriefed Ashley as best as she could.

Ashley felt confident, in her capacity as a consulting engineer, that she could successfully address her client's needs. And they made a strong team, these two. Nkasi knew about doing business in Nigeria. She had studied riparian law and water rights. Ashley, thoroughly trained in the mechanics of the device, had three years of experience in the field. "He who brings water, brings life," a representative of the Water Authority told her when they contracted her company's services. She was anxious to take her place at the table.

Early in the morning, after a fitful night's sleep, Ashley stepped out of the guest room and onto the cool tiles of the bathroom floor. She sat on the commode, rubbed her eyes, and then reached behind herself to flush. But nothing happened, nothing at all. She stood, finding the waste clumped in a small pool of water in the bottom of the bowl. She placed her hands under the tap on the sink, turned the cold and the hot knobs simultaneously, but no water ran from the faucet. She pulled back the curtain of the shower stall, placed a hand on the shiny metal, and turned. Air moved through the valve in response, but still no water.

"My cistern must have gone dry," Nkasi explained with a shrug. "I'd hoped it would last for your visit."

By evening the toilet was full of human waste, Ashley's face was grimy, her hands were tacky, and the crevices of her teeth felt cruddy. The hardest part was her thirst. Nkasi offered Ashley orange Fanta to drink throughout the day, but the sugary soda only made her thirst worse. By the next morning, when the water still didn't flow, Ashley was in tears.

Nkasi reached for the refrigerator and took out a container of water. "Here. I can offer you this," she said, extending the container to her guest, and explaining that she'd filled the bottle the nights before with premium-grade water from her tap, in preparation for her visit. Ashley took it and headed back toward the bathroom, saying, "That was so thoughtful. Thank you, Nkasi!"

"No, no!" she called to Ashley. "Bring that water back to the kitchen! I paid good money for that. It's for drinking only. No brushing teeth or washing face or hands or flat, greasy hair with that water!"

I didn't mean to offend you, thought Nkasi.

I am sorry, too. I just didn't understand, Ashley returned.

Maneuvering through the traffic proved more difficult than Nkasi had anticipated. It took them nearly 2 hours to travel only 20 kilometers. The problem was not so much with the cars but with the crowds. Throngs of people walked in the middle of the street . . . people everywhere, yelling and shouting.

"What's all this about?" Ashley asked.

"What did you expect?" Nkasi replied. "What did you think you'd find in coming here? We are in a state of emergency."

The two continued for a while without speaking, not even sharing *telepathoughts*. Suddenly, a loud thud shook the car.

"Lock your door!" Nkasi yelled.

"It *is* locked!" Ashley returned.

"Then, quick, get down on the floor so you won't be noticed!" She slid down onto the floor mat, her voice hushed and trembling. Chilled and sweating, a wave of nausea overcame Ashley.

The car shuddered from the force of the fists pounding and feet stomping on its trunk. People had climbed on top of their vehicle. Nkasi grabbed Ashley's hand and squeezed as the horde lifted their car onto two wheels. The rising volume of the shouting filled the air with chaos and confusion.

"They are demanding we get out," Nkasi explained calmly, "or they will turn the car over and smash the windows."

"Are you sure we should?" Ashley asked.

"Yes. But don't say a word, no matter what. I will do the talking for both of us." Increasingly weak and dizzy Ashley sensed she may soon need a bathroom.

Nkasi opened the door. Quickly, Ashley grabbed her bag from under the seat. The car was placed back down on its four wheels and both women were escorted out. A crowd of angry people surrounded them.

I don't understand what's happening. I don't understand the language they are speaking. I don't know what they are saying. Nkasi, what's going on?! Ashley's mind threw out in a panic.

I recognize this language as a dialect of my tribe. They represent one of the insurgencies that formed in opposition to the Water Authority. They are angry over the failing negotiations. Nkasi meant to keep Ashley calm and clear.

But we are on our way to help! Nkasi, tell them that. And tell them that we carry with us the solution to these problems, feeling anything but calm.

Nkasi tried to address the shouting men and women. But no one seemed to be listening. Four uniformed men arrived carrying rifles. The crowd drew back and settled down. One of them addressed Nkasi in English. She replied, gesturing emphatically as she relayed the urgency of getting to the negotiations. She explained that she was accompanied by a woman who came to Lagos from the U.S. with critical knowledge of how to build a device for extracting water from humidity. As the man spoke again Nkasi stood still, sullen as she listened. She was visibly shaken, her head turning from side to side, her arms clutched tightly around her abdomen.

What is it? Why are you so upset? Tell me what's happening, Nkasi. Ashley is hit with another wave of nausea.

"Someone infiltrated the municipal water works and deposited a biotoxin chemical into the premium-water system," Nkasi explained to Ashley. "One of the sensors detected its presence and released titanium dioxide to detoxify it. But the treatment didn't have the intended effect, so the entire water delivery system automatically went down. Water stopped flowing to community distribution centers. Now the negotiations are stalled and likely to fail. Civil war is sure to break out." Ashley tightened her hold on the bag with the device.

Once they see how efficiently this works to convert humidity to water, then everything will be OK.

I pray that you are right, my friend.

The way was cleared, and the pair was led into the open-air structure where the proceedings were being held. Chairs were arranged auditorium style, facing a platform at the front. Fans twirled slowly from the ceiling, barely moving the dense, hot air. Every seat was taken, and many stood in the aisles and along the exterior of the platform that held the structure. Men in jackets and women wearing skirts and blouses were seated facing the crowd. Everyone seemed to be talking at the same time, and the chaos was overwhelming. Ashley looked around, in search of a bathroom, finding no place for relief. Nkasi places a palm across Ashley's forehead. Something was very wrong. "You're running a high fever," Nkasi said with a frown. "I am so sorry," she whispered, "I didn't anticipate that the water would be poisoned."

Suddenly a man grabbed hold of Ashley. "Please come with me now!" he said in a panic. Ashley held fast to the device-containing bag. "It seems we've arrived just in time!" Nkasi whispered as she escorted her to the podium.

"Here is an engineer who has come from the U.S. She has something very important to share!" Nkasi announced into the microphone at the podium. The shouting lessened somewhat.

Ashley began to shake. She lifted the device from its container, handling it with great care, given both its delicacy and its value. She removed the shiny object and also a cup, which she placed beneath its spout. A hush comes over the room. With widened eyes the people grew still, leaning forward in their chairs. The wait was less than half a minute before clear water began to stream. Nkasi rushed forward, grabbing her companion in celebration. Ashley opened her mouth, and the vomit gushed out.

Chapter 6

Adult Stem Cells to Cure Diabetes-Induced Vision Loss

Shayn Peirce-Cottler

*Department of Biomedical Engineering and Department of Ophthalmology,
University of Virginia, PO Box 800759, Health System, Charlottesville,
VA 22908, USA*
shayn@virginia.edu

Diabetes is becoming a worldwide epidemic, and it is a complex disease that creates serious complications in nearly every tissue and organ. The eye is particularly susceptible to diabetes because it has so many blood vessels and is so metabolically active. Diabetic retinopathy (DR)—the manifestation of diabetes in the retina—is a leading cause of blindness in adults. Of all the different complications of diabetes that a patient will experience throughout his or her lifetime, DR is one of the first problems that they will face.

In the early stages of the disease, microaneurysms, balloon-like swellings in small areas of the retina's tiny blood vessels, occur. As the disease progresses, more and more blood vessels become dysfunctional, depriving the retina of crucial blood supply. Although the body grows new blood vessels to try

Creating Life from Life: Biotechnology and Science Fiction
Edited by Rosalyn W. Berne
Copyright © 2015 Pan Stanford Publishing Pte. Ltd.
ISBN 978-981-4463-58-4 (Hardcover), 978-981-4463-59-1 (eBook)
www.panstanford.com

to compensate for the loss, these neovessels are fragile and abnormal, tending to leak blood and plasma (edema). This vicious cycle causes more swelling and vision loss, fibrosis and eventual vessel dropout, and ultimately blindness resulting from retinal detachment (i.e., when the retinal tissue tears or rips away from the back wall of the eye that it is normally attached to).

Worldwide 347 million people have diabetes (Danaei et al., 2011). DR alone afflicts an estimated 101 million people worldwide, with a prevalence of 155 million expected by 2030 (Yau et al., 2012). DR is the leading cause of early-onset blindness and develops in 100% of type 1 and 60% of type 2 diabetic patients within 20 years of diagnosis. Diabetic macular edema associated with DR leads to vision loss in almost 30% of affected individuals within 20 years of disease inception in type 1 and type 2 patients (Cogan, Toussaint, and Kuwabara, 1961). While the pathogenesis and timing that underlie the condition will vary, always they involve destabilization of the retinal microvasculature. Microvascular abnormalities are some of the earliest pathologies associated with diabetes, setting the stage for later complications and disability.

More than 12,000 patients become blind each year due to ocular complications from DR. A long, steady progression of DR over many years, advancing from early nonproliferative changes to late proliferative disease, presents multiple opportunities and time points for therapeutic intervention. Although tight blood glucose control is the only preventative measure for DR, even with optimal control, retinopathy eventually develops. As the disease progresses there are procedures for restoring some vision function, such as laser surgery. And vitrectomy can be used to remove and replace the vitreous gel that has become clouded with blood that has escaped from the leaky, pathological retinal vessels. However, lasers destroy parts of the retina and peripheral vision, in particular. And eye injections of saline to replace the vitreous gel have to be done regularly over the course of one's life. A Food and Drug Administration

(FDA)-approved drug manufactured by Genentech, called Lucentis®, is widely used by ophthalmologists to treat DR and has been shown to reduce edema, but patients require monthly injections of the drug.

Retinal pericytes, cells that wrap around the endothelial cells that form capillaries—the smallest blood vessels in the retina—play a key role in capillary stabilization (Herman and D'Amore, 1985). Pericytes are likely to be amongst the first cellular casualties of diabetes in the eye. Death or dysfunction of pericytes, for reasons that are not well understood, lead to inadequate pericyte coverage of capillaries. Without pericytes supporting them, capillaries become disorganized and dysfunctional or are lost altogether. Once this happens in the diabetic eye, the pathological responses discussed above spiral out of control, and vision gradually declines, while the risk of blindness increases. There is currently no method to heal or regenerate blood vessels in the retina. What hope might there be, if any, for stopping the progression of this disease and reversing this path toward blindness?

The Role of Regenerative Medicine

While there are ongoing efforts to develop a bionic eye that could help restore a patient's vision, our efforts are focused on tapping into the body's built-in regenerative capabilities by using adult stem cells to heal the diseased retinal vasculature. Diabetic retinopathy (DR), a disease that proceeds over many years from initial pericyte dysfunction to microvascular degeneration, may be particularly well suited for stem cell–based therapies.

There are many different sources of stem cells, but we have chosen to focus on an adult stem cell population that can be pulled out of fat, or adipose, tissue (Chen et al., 2009). Stem cells obtained from fat, termed "adipose-derived stem cells," or ASCs for short, possess numerous benefits over other types of stem cells (Gimble et al., 2007). First, they are readily available and easily obtainable through routine liposuction procedures. Second, they are available in abundant quantities—a single liter of fat has hundreds of millions of stem cells. Third, ASCs can be cultured in the laboratory, frozen, and stored for later use, and their ability to differentiate into different types of cells—for example, muscle, bone, cartilage, and vascular cells—is retained. Fourth, and perhaps most importantly, these adult stem cells do not have the ethical concerns associated with embryonic stem cells.

Over the past decade, we and other scientists have established that when injected into an injured tissue or organ, ASCs can play a direct role in supporting the microvasculature, much like the native pericytes. We are now pursuing a new paradigm for treating DR that deploys ASCs to directly supplement (or replace) damaged retinal pericytes and restore a state of normalcy (homeostasis) in the retina.

In preclinical models, we have evaluated the extent to which human ASCs can be efficiently delivered to the retina through intravitreal pars plana injection into the vitreous (Mendel et al., 2013). We have shown the injected cells reach the retina, and many of them find their way to the retinal blood vessels and start to look and behave like the native pericytes—aligning with and enwrapping the microvessels and expressing proteins on their cell membranes that are indicative of a pericyte phenotype. Our data also supports that ASCs have a functionally beneficial impact on the diseased blood vessels in the eye. Their presence prevents both capillary dropout and pathological blood vessel growth. Functional stabilization of retinal vasculature by ASCs, even in areas of the retina where no direct incorporation of ASC progenitors on retinal vessels is observed, suggests that ASCs can also exert their therapeutic effects simply by producing and secreting health-inducing proteins. Together, these results suggest that injected ASCs may assist in stabilizing retinal microvasculature that is otherwise acutely unstable.

Further work is clearly needed before the preclinical successes demonstrated by ASC therapy for DR can move into clinical practice. For example, it is important to explore the extent to which injected ASCs may help maintain or restore normal function of the native pericyte population in the face of persistent toxic environments, such as chronic hyperglycemia. (Injecting ASCs into the eye will not, after all, cure the patient of diabetes.) Given the ASCs' ability to survive the relatively greater hypoxic conditions of adipose tissue as compared to the eye, they may be particularly well suited to respond to such insults. Moreover, not all fat is created equal. We know that the age, overall health, specific fat depots, and possibly gender of the fat donor can impact the ability of the ASCs to provide a therapeutic benefit. The extent to which the therapeutic potential of ASCs harvested from diabetic patients compares to that of ASCs harvested from healthy patients is an important consideration when strategizing an autologous or allogeneic therapy.

Despite the remaining work required to translate ASC stem cell therapy to the clinic, experimental results suggest that stem cell–based strategies for retinal vasculopathies may one day allow a shift in focus from destructive laser treatment of late-stage DR to earlier preventative interventions aimed at stabilizing existing retinal microvasculature. The consistent and robust microvascular-stabilizing properties of ASC-derived pericytes offer hope that such a regenerative treatment for retinal vasculopathies, including DR, may be attainable.

Acknowledgments

Financial support from the National Institutes of Health through R01 EY022063-01 and from the University of Virginia Launchpad Fund created by Paul and Diane Manning is gratefully acknowledged. Coprincipal investigators on the research project include Dr. Paul A. Yates, MD, PhD (University of Virginia, Department of Ophthalmology) and Dr. Ira M. Herman, PhD (Tufts University). Other key contributors include Dr. Adam Katz, MD (University of Florida) and Dr. Elizabeth Rakoczy (University of Western Australia). Student and trainee contributors include Tom Mendel (project leader), Stephen Cronk, David Kao, Erin Clabough, Tatiana Demidova-Rice, Jennifer Durham, Brendan Zotter, and Scott Seaman.

References

Chen, C. W., Montelatici, E., Crisan, M., Corselli, M., Huard, J., Lazzari, L., and Péault, B. 2009). Perivascular multi-lineage progenitor cells in human organs: regenerative units, cytokine sources or both? *Cytokine Growth Factor Review*, 20, 429–434. doi:http://dx.doi.org/10.1016/j.cytogfr.2009.10.014.

Cogan, D. G., Toussaint, D., and Kuwabara, T. (1961). Retinal vascular patterns. IV. Diabetic retinopathy. *Archives of Ophthalmology*, 66, 366–378. doi:http://dx.doi.org/10.1001/archopht.1961.00960010368014.

Danaei, G., Finucane, M. M., Lu, Y., Singh, G. M., Cowan, M. J., Paciorek, C. J., . . . and Ezzati, M. (2011). National, regional, and global trends in fasting plasma glucose and diabetes prevalence since 1980: systematic analysis of health examination surveys and epidemiological studies with 370 country-years and 2.7 million participants. *Lancet*, 378(9785) 31–40.

Gimble, J. M., Katz, A. J., and Bunnell, B. A. (2007). Adipose-derived stem cells for regenerative medicine. *Circulation Research*, 100, 1249–1260.

Herman, I. M., and D'Amore, P. A. (1985). Microvascular pericytes contain muscle and nonmuscle. *Journal of Cell Biology*, 101, 43–52. doi:http://dx.doi.org/10.1083/jcb.101.1.43.

Mendel, T. A., Clabough, E. B., Kao, D. S., Demidova-Rice, T. N., Durham, J. T., Zotter, B. C., . . . and Yates, P. A. (2013) Pericytes derived from adipose-derived stem cells protect against retinal vasculopathy. *PLOS One*, 8(5), e65691. doi:10.1371/journal.pone.0065691.

Yau, J. W., Rogers, S. L., Kawasaki, R., Lamoureux, E. L., Kowalski, J. W., Bek, T., . . . and Wong, T. Y. Meta-Analysis for Eye Disease (META-EYE) Study Group. (2012). Global prevalence and major risk factors of diabetic retinopathy. *Diabetes Care*, 35, 556–564. doi:10.2337/dc11-1909.

Shadows and Sugars and Shades of Gray (Madeline, Part 2)

Rosalyn W. Berne

M ADELINE STIRRED SLUGGISHLY FROM another poor night's sleep. How many times had she gotten up to pee? Three, four, more?

The morning's light peered through the blinds on her bedroom's triple-hung windows. "Open wide," she commanded. The yellow rays hit her eyelids with a jolt as the blinds turned upward in unison. Normally they'd lift automatically at 7:00 a.m., but these days Madeline preferred to use the voice command setting; she never knew what time she'd have the will to get up. She'd felt so tired for the last few months. Or was it a whole year she'd been sleepy throughout the day? She squinted, rubbing her eyes to try to clear her vision.

"Forget it," Madeline mumbled. "I definitely need some more sleep."

She turned over on her side, pulling the blankets over her head. Moaning, she closed her eyes again. Madeline was neither awake nor asleep, so she just lay there thinking, *Who am I? What have I become? Who occupies this body? Something feels unfamiliar.*

A while later, she didn't know exactly how long, the sound of snoring woke her.

"Oh my!" It was nearly 10:00 a.m. "That must have been me."

Madeline tossed the covering aside and opened her eyes. Her job started at 11:00 a.m. Being there on time would require getting up right away. She felt alert but not rested yet eager to move along. An odd sense of vulnerability made her feel nervous. Something wasn't quite right.

She sat up, reaching for the glass of orange juice she'd placed on her bed stand the night before. Oddly, it was only half full. "Or is it half empty?" she snickered. She sipped the delightful drink with satisfaction, as she tried to recall her evening ritual: poured the chilled juice into a 16-ounce tumbler (her favored one of hand-blown glass made in Italy); headed for the bedroom with the glass in hand; glanced back to be certain the kitchen, dining area, den, and hall lights had all turned themselves off; put the drink down on the nightstand; entered the bathroom; used the toilet, washed her face, brushed her teeth, and combed her hair; and got into bed, told the blinds to close, told the music to play, and finally fell asleep.

"No, that's not right. That's not how it went last night."

She took sips of orange juice right before the bedroom lights were dimmed. That explained the reduced volume of juice this morning.

She slurped the last of the tepid liquid. At least for the moment, it seems to quench her incessant thirst. She placed her feet on the floor and grimaced a bit over the tenderness. The sores were getting worse.

Heading for the bathroom to take her morning shower, Madeline delighted in her independence. No one needed to help her out of bed, guide her into the tub, or help her wash her body. Her days of extreme obesity were over, although maybe it would be prudent to determine her actual weight and stick more closely to the prescribed regimen. Her stomach seemed larger than a few weeks ago. Some of her clothing no longer fit the way it once did.

Moving with relative agility, she removed clean undergarments from the chest of drawers, took the tartan plaid wool pants and red cardigan sweater down from their hangers in the closet, and dressed herself. She put on her shoes very carefully to minimize the pain. New clothing. How nice. Each and every item, including coats, boots, and shoes, all purchased for Madeline by the Foundation. They'd assured her before they performed the procedure that any personal effects would be provided for, along with a generous stipend. How grateful. How wonderful. How very thoughtful of them. Of course, it wasn't a one-way street; she had been a help to them, too, as a subject of their novel research.

Madeline walked out of Unit 111, as was her regular daily routine, and made her way down the two flights of steps, along the walkways, past the shrubs, and into the community courtyard. These days she was paid for the time she spent there, employed as the playground attendant. The well-being of the community's children during their mandatory outdoor playtime was now *her* responsibility.

Madeline took a seat on the bench, placed her lunch sack next to her side, and picked up the device she'd been given to document playground activity. Yes, there were cameras installed, revealing every square inch of the community's outdoor spaces. And records were automatically kept through those recordings. But residents decided they liked having a real person observing. And since she was there anyway, why not pay Madeline? Who else? She knew every one of the children by name, what they looked like, and whom they played with. What a perfect match.

Madeline took note of the activity, considering which details to include in her report. How about the lyrics of the songs the girls sang as they jumped rope and played hopscotch? Or the pranks the boys planned when they gathered together in tight circles under the trees? Madeline decided yes, because based on her experience, everything had significance. Physical activity was helpful and good, but play became more engaging when it included singing and joking and gossip. These may be valuable notations for future consideration regarding mandatory outdoor play.

Obesity had become an epidemic. Vigilance was required in the children's health.

Madeline spoke softly into the small device held at her mouth so as not to draw attention to herself. Dictating the names and activities, she hoped her words were transmitted accurately:

- *Shawna jumps for 10 minutes and turns the ropes for 20. She moves slower than she might and lifts her feet only enough to clear the ropes. Higher lifts would improve her metabolism.*
- *Ben just sits moping about, wanting his blue box. As it turns out, he's hidden the device in his pants and has furtively been watching a cartoon that is projected onto his sunglasses.*
- *Nathaniel is chasing the girls. I let it be because they seem to enjoy it. But when the girls turn on him, chasing him into a corner, Nathaniel starts to cry. Reminder to self: Best leave the boy to sort it out on his own.*

As the days went by, spring shifting into summer, Madeline came to depend more and more on her hearing and to some extent on her sense of smell. Touch was important, too, though most of the children didn't like it when she patted them on the head or tried to take hold of their hands. Fortunately, each child's voice was distinctive, and each girl and boy had a distinguishing scent.

The degeneration was rapid and frightening. Each day the obscurities grew more severe. The seesaw no longer appeared as a straight board . . . more like a puzzle piece with jagged edges. The chains on the swing set were as squiggly lines, their movements obscured by odd shapes. Looking up was just as disorienting. Clouds, no longer white puffs, or streaks of light gray, had become ugly patchworks of darkness against the sky.

And the grass, walkways, and stairs under her feet became a complex, changing maze as she walked.

On the Saturday morning that Madeline tripped, climbing out of the bathtub, the sensors set off alarms. The cameras captured the image of her body as she lay writhing in pain on the tile floor. Help arrived within just a few minutes. The diagnosis was made right away. "Type two," they called it as they read the analysis. "You mean I have 'sugar'?" Madeline asked in dismay, using the term her grandmother had called her own condition. Fortunately, the Foundation would help her. Placing nanobots in her blood, which would release sugar at optimal levels, would also monitor the insulin. As for the degeneration of the macula, her eyes could be removed and replaced by ones grown in the optics production facilities.

Madeline refused the intervention. One major procedure was enough for a lifetime. Plus, she was still making adjustments to her new body. She insisted she would be fine and said no to further Foundation care. Though that night was a painful one for her, Madeline returned to the playground the very next day.

Only three children came out for mandatory play that Sunday, the others being on vacation or away at summer camp. Madeline took notes of the relative normality of the activity, enjoying the sounds of their joyful engagements. Until, that is, Madeline began to sense her stomach tightening with trepidation. Though her senses tried to tell her, she didn't realize what was happening when Caroline slipped off the jungle gym. Madeline didn't make out that the child had fallen down. Her little body made no sound when it hit the rubber matting or when the bones in her tiny neck snapped. She didn't even cry out in pain.

Caroline was the last child out playing that day, the other two having gone back inside. So no one was there to report that Caroline was lying still, and unconscious, on the ground. Of course, the cameras had recorded the entire mishap, but rarely did anyone bother to take note. The monitors mounted in the interior common spaces of the residences played unattended and unobserved.

Madeline looked upward, to the overcast sky, seeing broken patches of white and gray. She looked straight ahead and side to side, noting how still the shadows had become. She looked at the pavement, the clay, and the grass and then noticed the small lizard-like shape. On second thought, it looked more like a turtle, with its feet pulled up under its shell. Madeline heard it breathing.

"Caroline?!" she called out, lunging from the bench, approaching the blob in sheer terror.

It wasn't her fault that Caroline fell. Thankfully through regeneration of the vertebrae and severed cord, Caroline regained her mobility. But the entire affair was enough to cause Madeline to reconsider. What if she'd seen it coming? Could she possibly have prevented the fall? What if she'd realized right away what had happened? Would the damage have been less severe? She knew what she had to do.

The optical procedure was uneventful. Her replacement eyes functioned well. As a medical case Madeline's was straightforward. With the bots coursing through her veins, her insulin levels were internally monitored and stabilized.

Mandatory outdoor playtime continued through the winter months. Madeline was there every day. The children found ways to be creative out in the cold and snow and were especially fun to watch.

Notes:

- *Clem uses shiny silver tubes for the snow-bot's nose and the eyes. I wonder where he found those. I hope they are safe for play.*

— *Sarah likes to make snow angels, but Doug insists on messing them up.*

— *Caroline avoids the jungle gym, preferring only to swing.*

Madeline found herself thinking about that nice man, the one who'd moved into the community last spring. Too bad she didn't catch his name or which unit he was living in. When she'd thought of him now and then, it was notable how her heart rate would increase. Each day as she observed the children play, she found herself hoping he might come by. It was April when finally he did.

"Hi, there!" said the professor, taking a seat on the bench.

"Oh, hi!" Madeline replied. "I haven't seen you since last spring. How've you been?"

The man explained about how busy things had gotten with his new position. How the research was taking up most of his time. He spoke of the pressure to get out publications and why that meant little time to relax and socialize.

"You must be really devoted to your work," she commented.

"Yes, but as I passed through the courtyard and saw you today, I decided perhaps I needed mandatory outdoor time, too!"

Madeline chuckled over his saying that as she studied the lines of his face. Something about him was different. The shape of his mouth, the placement of his nose, the way his chin sat square on his face, the scaly features of his pale, pink skin . . . Seeing with her newly replaced eyes, he wasn't that appealing after all.

Chapter 7

Neogenesis

Reginald H. Garrett

Department of Biology, Physical Life Sciences Building (PLSB),
University of Virginia, 90 Geldard Drive, Charlottesville, VA 22903, USA
rhg@virginia.edu

> *In the beginning God created the heaven and the*
> *earth. And the earth was without form, and void; and*
> *darkness was upon the face of the deep.*
>
> (Genesis 1:1, 2)

In May 2010, scientists at the J. Craig Venter Institute (JCVI) reported the creation of the first self-replicating synthetic bacterial cell. This achievement was touted as the latest step toward creating life from scratch and "a defining moment in the history of biology" (Pennisi, 2010). The genome synthesized was that of *Mycoplasma mycoides*, a bacterium that causes respiratory infections in cows and goats. Mycoplasma are among the simplest of bacteria. The mycoplasma genome is just over a million base pairs of DNA (versus 3 billion in humans). What the JCVI researchers (Gibson et al., 2010) actually accomplished

Creating Life from Life: Biotechnology and Science Fiction
Edited by Rosalyn W. Berne
Copyright © 2015 Pan Stanford Publishing Pte. Ltd.
ISBN 978-981-4463-58-4 (Hardcover), 978-981-4463-59-1 (eBook)
www.panstanford.com

was the assembly of pieces of chemically synthesized DNA that collectively comprise the genome of *Mycoplasma mycoides.*

Appreciation of DNA as the material of heredity is virtually universal, to the point where it is commonly used in pronouncements describing an attribute someone might have, such as "playing the saxophone is in his DNA." And many are aware that DNA is composed of two strands of nucleic acid that wrap around each other to form a double helix. Fewer people concern themselves with the details; let's summarize them here, to connect DNA structure with its pre-eminent function as a carrier of information. Each strand is a polymer of chemical units called nucleotides. In turn, each nucleotide consists of a ring of carbon and nitrogen atoms; these rings are termed "bases" in the language of chemistry. Each base is attached to a sugar that has five carbon atoms. Four of the five carbons and one oxygen from the sugar form a ring structure as well, and the fifth carbon atom from the sugar is linked to another group of atoms called a phosphate. The phosphate group consists of one phosphorus and four oxygen atoms. The phosphate atoms allow the sugar rings to join up with one another to form a polymer of nucleotides, or polynucleotide. Nucleic acids are polynucleotides. When polynucleotides form, the sugar–phosphate array is the backbone of the polymer and the bases, one per nucleotide, project above the backbone. A good analogy for a polynucleotide might be a strand of Christmas tree lights, with the sugar–phosphate backbone as the "wire" and the bases as "lightbulbs." In such an analogy, there are just four "colors" of "bulbs," or four different base/ring structures, which, in DNA language, are referred to by A, C, G, and T, from the first letters of their names, adenine, cytosine, guanine, and thymine. A defining feature of DNA as genetic material is that in the double helix of two polynucleotide strands, each base in one strand is paired with a base in the other strand, and the rule of pairing is absolute: An A in one strand is always paired with a T in the other strand and vice versa; similarly, a C in one strand is always paired with a G in the other strand and vice versa. Thus, if you know the sequence of bases along one strand, you automatically know the sequence along the other. And this is the basis of life—the sequence of bases represents the digital information to make an organism, encoded as the order of A, C, G, and T bases along a DNA strand. The other strand, the partner to this strand, called the complementary strand, has the same information content, as embedded in the A–T and C–G pairing rule. Defining the size of DNA molecules in terms of the number of base pairs (bp), or indicating the information content of genomes in terms of the number of base pairs, follows logically.

What did the JCVI researchers really do? They bought 1,078 strands of DNA from a biotechnology company that specializes in the chemical synthesis of DNA molecules with any desired sequence of A, C, G, and T bases. Call such a company on the phone, or better yet, send it an email, and it will respond with the nucleic acid molecule you desire, for a price. (Safeguards are in place to prevent anyone from ordering the AIDS virus genome, the anthrax genome, or any other DNA sequence that might be used for nefarious purposes.) Each purchased molecule was 1,080 bp long, and when arranged in the proper order, the 1,078 molecules spelled out the genome of *Mycoplasma mycoides* (*M. mycoides*). The tricky part for the JCVI team was to put all these molecules together to form a single, circular DNA double helix with the unique *M. mycoides* gene sequence (bacterial genomes are circular). The scientists exploited well-known techniques of molecular biology to construct this circular genome within yeast cells, and then they purified the intact bacterial DNA circles from the yeast. What they had in hand then was a completely synthetic DNA genome for a specific organism. Another way of thinking about what they had is to realize, as we have noted, that the information encoded by the genome of an organism is basically a set of instructions for making that organism. In and of itself, it can do nothing. Like the letters on this or any other page, the information in DNA is, without some means to detect and decipher it, an inert array of characters. For the letters on this page, the means is the reader's eyes and mind. For DNA, it is the cytoplasm of a cell that is competent to access and express the information it encodes.

Mycoplasma capricolum (*M. capricolum*) cells, a species closely related to *M. mycoides*, were chosen as the recipients for the synthetic *M. mycoides* DNA. To ensure that the transplanted mycoides DNA had usurped control and was directing the activity of the host *M. capricolum* cells, the scientists had engineered "watermarks" into the synthetic DNA. Since these watermarks were found in the DNA of the manipulated mycoplasma cells recovered after many rounds of cell division and multiplication, it was proof that these cells had been transformed from *M. capricolum* cells into a new form of life directed by a synthetic genome. The watermarks were based on imaginative use of several consecutive A, C, G, and/or T bases to encrypt the letters of the alphabet so that three great quotations from recent human history were encoded:

> To live, to err, to fall, to triumph, to recreate life out of life.
> —James Joyce

> See things not as they are, but as they might be.
> —J. Robert Oppenheimer (as cited in *American Prometheus*, his biography by Kai Bird and Martin J. Sherwin)

> What I cannot build, I cannot understand.
> —Richard Feynman (Saenz, 2010, reveals how these messages were encoded.)

The scientists dubbed their new organism "Synthia." J. Craig Venter, founder of the JCVI, is seeking a patent for JCV-SYN 1.0, the code name for Synthia. As Venter has noted many times (see, e.g., Alstrom, 2012), these experiments were meant as a proof of principle, to demonstrate that it is possible to type out a synthetic genome, synthesize it chemically, and express it in an appropriate cell cytoplasm. At one level, this is indeed neogenesis, the creation of new life. Indeed, nothing exactly like Synthia ever existed before. Going on from this point, it is apparent that treating the DNA of an organism as a software program easily amenable to enhancements opens a vast possibility not only for the biosynthesis of rare chemicals and new drugs but also for the creation of engineered microorganisms capable of producing biofuels or remediating oil spills or toxic waste sites—a veritable neogenesis of organisms designed for some purpose. Further speculation leads to *transhumanism*, the directed manipulation of the human genome to produce humans with desired traits, such as a higher muscle-to-fat ratio, resistance to a certain disease, or even improved cognition.

DNA as information also promises to be an extremely efficient data storage device. As described by George Church and Ed Regis in *Regenesis* (Church and Regis, 2012), the Massachusetts Institute of Technology established an intercollegiate genetically engineered machines (iGEM) competition in 2004. Imaginative undergraduates around the world have come up with some astounding creations, and each year, a jamboree is held to judge entries. In 2010, a group of students from the Chinese University of Hong Kong described their goal of turning the common intestinal bacterium (and lab organism), *Escherichia coli (E. coli)*, into a data storage system. Their scheme encoded, encrypted, and stored the text of our *Declaration of Independence* in engineered *E. coli* cells in a form that could be retrieved. Any form of encoded information—music, pictures, and video—can be encoded and stored as DNA; the technology currently exists.

Google estimates that the total number of books ever written is 130 million. Longish books, of the length of *Moby Dick* or *Harry Potter and the Order of the Phoenix*, contain about 1 million characters (letters and spaces). Taking these books as representative (thus erring on the high side), 130 trillion (130×10^{12}) characters represents an overestimate of the total written text accumulated over the full span of human history. At 6 billion characters (bp) of DNA information per human cell, all the words of humanity could be encrypted and stored in the DNA within several thousand cells. (Since a relatively small portion of human DNA carries information that is useful to the cell, this notion is not so far fetched.) A rough estimate for the weight of a single human cell is 10^{-9} g, so a few micrograms (10^{-6} g) of tissue would be sufficient to contain this information. Of course, a great deal of redundancy would be desirable, since errors do occur in data storage and transmission. Even with many thousand-fold redundancy, a small bit of tissue (a wart?) could hold all of history. Now that information can be readily encoded within DNA, spy stories about purloined state secrets encoded on microfilm or in microchips seem old fashioned and trite. How will governments and industries ever discover a stolen secret encoded as DNA?

References

Alstrom, D. (2012, July 12). Venter says "synthetic life is coming." *The Irish Times*.

Church, G. E., and Regis, E. (2012). *Regenesis*. New York, NY: Basic Books.

Gibson, D. G., Glass, J. I., Lartigue, C., Noskov, V. N., Chuang, R.-Y., Algire, M. A., . . . and Venter, J. C. (2010). Creation of a bacterial cell controlled by a chemically synthesized genome. *Science*, **329**, 52–56.

Pennisi, E. (2010). Synthetic genome brings new life to bacterium. *Science*, **328**, 958–959.

Saenz, A. (2010). Secret messages coded into DNA of Venter synthetic bacteria, http://singularityhub.com/2010/05/24/venters-newest-synthetic-bacteria-has-secret-messages-coded-in-its-dna/.

Madness Enough to Break the World

WHAT DOES GOD HAVE left to offer that man has not seized for himself? It is a tricky question, and probably not best pondered while overseeing a heavily armed robot flying thousands of feet above Uzbekistan. Warriors as far back as World War I have described combat as interminable boredom punctuated by moments of sheer terror. In the trenches the boredom could easily spread out over months, and then hell consumes all for just a few moments. In the silence that follows, men have often discovered God, either in person or at a distance. While many deep insights into human nature and the systems of the world have their origins in these deep and deadly silences, they are discovered in hindsight. Combat did not lend itself to philosophical musings in the moment. It wasn't until the new model of warfare was discovered in the 21st century that man came to appreciate the divinity of the action at a distance centuries of bloody innovation had created. Perhaps now, the seconds of sheer terror were precisely the moment in which the divine perpetrator should contemplate most fully its own power.

The world below, an ugly *bricolage* of postindustrial waste and desperate attempts to wring sustenance from the sparse watershed of the North Nuratau Mountains, seemed incredibly vulnerable. The Angel of Death circled overhead, the focus of its evolving pylon turn a sad little convoy of Soviet-era trucks on a mountain path. The drivers of the trucks probably felt a little

*Centre for the Study of the Sciences and the Humanities (SVT), Postboks 7805, 5020 Bergen, Norway. sean.hays@svt.uib.no

frightened by their own speed on that unpaved and crumbling road, but the scramble to reach Samarkand pushed caution aside. In the divine musings of operator UJ-532, they crawled pathetically along. The dust plume behind them seemed more dynamic and powerful than the trucks themselves.

The Operator (as UJ-532's console mates called him) received his third confirmation of clearance to engage and released the Hellfire. The display in front of him washed out for a second as the missile's engine ignited, and then the desert below returned on the other side of a fading shimmer of heat. He targeted the center truck in the convoy, gently nudging the targeting reticule to guide the ordnance home. The truck remained small on the screen for far too long and then grew with terrifying speed just before the feed cut to snow. Max's alternate targeting screens showed the thermobaric warhead detonating inside the truck, and the resulting pressure wave and fireball completely demolishing the vehicle and its passengers. The lead and follow trucks were close enough to the target to be thrown through the air, and it is unlikely that any passengers survived. He confirmed that the target had been destroyed, though it seemed unnecessary, as the White House was watching the same feeds he was. "Mr. President . . . " the Secretary of Defense began, but he was quickly cut off by the Commander in Chief.

"Just give me a minute here, Charlie. This is not exactly our finest hour."

The SecDef took a breath, "I understand, Mr. President, when you are ready, sir."

Watching these strikes was always an unpleasant experience for the president, but today was a uniquely difficult operation, and he seemed visibly older than when he entered the room. The campaign and his six years in office had turned a vibrant man in the prime of his life into a gray-haired gentleman with a dignified but weary affect.

"OK, Charlie, sorry for the interruption. Let's hear it." The other members of the cabinet stared down at the table, frozen in place.

"Yes, Mr. President, we have subjects one and two in custody. Subject three was in the truck targeted by today's op. We chose to use thermobarics to ensure the subject's payload was incinerated. It is extremely unlikely that any residual data will be recovered from the wreckage, but we have secured clearance from our counterpart in-country to insert a recovery team and mop up."

Despite the president's distaste for this sort of thing, it was usually best to just tear the bandage off as quickly and efficiently as possible, but this time he almost seemed to wince every time the SecDef referred to "subjects" and incineration. His face became decidedly sour at the mention of a payload. The president looked as if an invisible hand was forcing him down into a chair that was suddenly comically too large for him.

"Mr. President, it is with deepest regret that I have to report that subjects four and five are still outside the pocket. You have the latest all-source intelligence summary in your briefing packet. The CIA places four in Suzhou, one of the endless suburbs surrounding Shanghai, and there is a high degree of confidence that the Chinese are already offloading his data. Subject five isn't even on the radar, but given his last contact it is safe to assume he is also in PRC custody. Mr. President, we are out of both time and options."

The SecDef paused, as the president had dropped his head into his hands. Time seemed to slow as the president's shoulders began to softly shake. He never imagined in all his years that he would see this man break, and wasn't prepared to admit to himself it was happening now. "Mr. President . . . sir, it's time." The president didn't even lift his head. He croaked, "Do it," from behind the screen of his fingers, like a child convinced that if he couldn't see evil, it could not see him.

It was dark in Shenyang, just a bit outside of Beijing. The police had implemented a curfew just before sundown. It had been done using brute manpower rather than setting up any obvious barricades or checkpoints. The city streets were nearly empty, as most of the officers were staying just inside homes and business, making only brief patrols to look for troublemakers. None of this was apparent to the frantic occupants of Site 17. The building was not externally labeled, and no name for it appeared on any maps. Seemingly benign bureaucrats normally occupied the floors above street level, but these levels were dark and empty tonight. The floors below ground could not be accessed from within the building or the street above. What appeared to be a massive storm outflow duct into an artificial river several miles away allowed vehicle access to the massive blast doors several stories under the streets. The complex then burrowed six more stories under the city. It was brightly lit, and the activity within was frantic.

Men and women in unmarked military uniforms hustled through the corridors, though they never actually ran. Instead it was a quick and determined walk, taking care to keep to the center of the corridors, which allowed them to notice one another coming around corners before any collisions could occur. Dr. Fang finished scrubbing out of the operating theater and prepared to enter the lab complex. The two were adjacent and had been purpose-built for this mission. The American subject in custody had already been questioned and then turned over to her for data extraction of a different sort. She had been a bit ashamed, as a professional, at the crude nature of the operation, which employed a machine not unlike a liposuction device to penetrate the subject's intestine and remove a large sample from within. He was still in the operating theater, strapped to a cruciform table in case they needed additional samples. Despite the ugliness of the procedure, she was fairly sure that they had what they needed.

A dozen technicians were quickly processing the sample and extracting a large host of bacteria. Most of it is bound to be the normal fauna resident in the human gut, which actually made her job a bit more difficult, as what she was looking for was a modified strain of *E. coli*, which will look and act much like the normal *E. coli* one would expect in the human digestive tract. The bacteria were being washed through various chemical mixtures, which would tag each strain individually. The tagged bacteria would then be subjected to DNA analysis. If all went as planned, it would not take particularly long to identify the watermarks included in the bugs the Americans had planted in this man's stomach. In "useless" segments of the DNA of the modified bacteria a series of obvious tags would be coded. Once she had located the proper strain, she could decode the DNA of many samples and then turn the resulting data strings over to the cryptanalysts from the Ministry of State Security (MSS). The American was persuaded to provide some clues as to how the data could be decrypted, and along with information from other sources it would not be long before the code was cracked.

Dr. Fang was prepared to head back to her flat for the night, perhaps spend some time with her fiancé, when one of the techs showed her a tagged sample. In the solution, under magnification, she could see crowds of what appeared to be thousands of tiny sausages. Mixed in among the bacteria were thousands of tiny cysts. The cysts were spiked, like cockleburs, and just a bit smaller than the *E. coli*. The cysts clung to the bacteria like the burs they resembled. She watched as several of them began to break apart, perhaps succumbing to the UV radiation from the laboratory lights. Dr. Fang continued to watch as the burs disintegrated, and within each was a tight bundle of matter, which, under higher magnification, resolved into bundles of round cells. The cells appeared to actually be icosahedral in shape and didn't show any immediate reaction to the *E. coli* bacteria in the sample. She watched for some time, and when nothing new developed she logged the information and then scrubbed out of the lab to head home. The MSS would contact her when the DNA information had been decrypted, and she could then get back to work. The American showed all of the phenotypic changes they had been told to expect from one of the modification subjects, and she was eager to get to work refining the inevitably crude American DNA syntheses and applying them to her own subjects, who were waiting in a second lab several levels below this one.

Her MSS liaison called at exactly 6:00 a.m. the next morning. The decryption could not possibly be complete, but they had an escort waiting outside her building. Dr. Fang felt anxiety creep into her chest and head, a frisson that tightened her core muscles and made her briefly lightheaded. Her fiancé remained in bed as she quickly dressed, tied her hair back, and headed down to the street. The men waiting on the street were in plain clothes, but their demeanor and the wire helices running out of their ears marked them as part of the security forces. The car they silently ushered her into was unmarked and discrete but had the sound and feel of an armored vehicle. She sat alone in the back, and the doors were locked from the front seats beyond a heavy partition. Her anxiety rose to the level of panic for a moment, and she began to review in her mind the events of the previous day, looking for the error she had made to warrant a visit like this one. A person of lower status within the military-industrial-educational complex in China might get a visit from the security services for almost any error at work, but she must have screwed up really badly.

The car went not to Site 17 but to another unmarked building on the other side of the city. The building was known by most to house the local offices of the MSS, and her car pulled through an automated gate into a secure underground garage. She was ushered to an elevator, which took her below ground several more stories. When she exited, Mr. Wei was waiting for her. He had several security toughs with him, and the look on his face was more grim than usual. He brusquely told her to remain silent and to follow him. He led the way into an interrogation suite where two men and a woman, all of whom appeared to be part of the technical staff, based on their physiques and dress, were waiting for them.

She sat alone on one side of a rectangular metal table, and Mr. Wei shoved a red folder across the table at her. The technical people busied themselves with their computers, which were physically wired into the building's secure network. In the folder was a report from the cryptanalysts, detailing the initial findings from the DNA decryption begun last night. The report also noted the information she had logged about the cysts and their icosahedral cargo. The *E. coli* strain contained enough "nonfunctioning" DNA to encrypt reams of technical data, which is what she had expected. Instead, they had so far located only a single message, repeated many times.

The American subjects had been intercepted attempting to get the data China believed to be encoded in the *E. coli* DNA carried in their guts to a Russian lab in Uzbekistan. A three-star general in the US Air Force had, according to their sources, arranged for the subjects to be smuggled out of the states to the Russian lab so that his ideological compatriots, Christian zealots in the Russian Orthodox Church, could put it to use in furtherance of their cause. The experiments the Americans had conducted created a set of five test subjects with extraordinary new capabilities. The subjects had broad immunity to a wide variety of very nasty diseases, along with radically increased metabolic efficiency allowing for sustained operations over many days without sleep or nourishment. The experiments had also increased density in all muscle fiber types, as well as enhancements to a variety of cognitive abilities. MSS human intelligence sources had discovered that the general had used technology from another set of experiments conducted by the air force to encrypt and encode the technical data from these experiments in the DNA of modified *E. coli* bacteria, which were introduced into the guts of the test subjects just prior to their being smuggled out of the country on a cargo flight bound for the AfPak theater of operations.

Since the saga had started some two years ago, China had been quietly creating the facilities necessary to extract the data itself, before the subjects could be delivered to the Russian lab. A massive network of scientists and security operatives had been assembled, along with a series of redundant, hardened sites with the requisite lab facilities. Test subjects had been selected from elite soldiers in various branches of the military, and now the whole network was tensely holding its breath, waiting for her. Dr. Fang read the sentence several times. She had been educated at US primary and secondary schools, her graduate studies had been conducted at Harvard, and her English was flawless, but the sentence just didn't make sense.

In the eye of an angry god, you will find madness enough to break the world.

The frisson she had felt earlier returned, stronger this time. She thought of the icosahedrons that had emerged from the cysts under the microscope last night and how much they appeared to be eyes. She thought of her fiancé, who had warmed dinner for her when she came home, and made love to her before they fell asleep in each other's arms. She had dreamed of her son, not yet conceived, and had been untroubled through the night.

It felt like an eternity passed before she realized she was staring up at the ceiling, having fallen from her chair. The sensation of a vibration and spasm in her chest and stomach would not leave her, and her limbs were rigid. Mr. Wei's face swam into view, and he was obviously yelling something at her, but she could not hear him over the pounding of her own heart. The modified herpes virus, those icosahedrons from her lab sample, invading her central nervous system disrupted her lower motor cortex and silenced even her thundering heart.

Chapter 8

Keys to Bioproducts from Agriculture

Elizabeth Hood

Arkansas Biosciences Institute and College of Agriculture and Technology,
Arkansas State University, AR 72467, USA
ehood@astate.edu

The world is changing. However, some things never change.
In different eras, changes are different, and the speed of those
changes also changes. For example, in the 1910s and 1920s, the
invention of cars changed the way we move, telephones allowed
us to talk to people without being in front of them, airplanes
allowed us to move quickly around the world, and, later in
the 1930s, refrigeration allowed us to eat food that wasn't
grown within 100 miles, like tomatoes in winter (unless you
live in Mexico)! Who among us does not now use a personal
or minicomputer or the web? However, similar technological
changes also made it possible to kill more people in wars, a
reminder that new technologies, although important and useful,
can also be used for destructive purposes. Nevertheless, we will
always be inventing, introducing, and using new technologies.
We can't imagine a world without electronics, and the youngest

Creating Life from Life: Biotechnology and Science Fiction
Edited by Rosalyn W. Berne
Copyright © 2015 Pan Stanford Publishing Pte. Ltd.
ISBN 978-981-4463-58-4 (Hardcover), 978-981-4463-59-1 (eBook)
www.panstanford.com

generation can't imagine (when it is old enough to reflect on it) a world without touchscreens and Facebook (Rosin, 2013)!

Oil is contributing to climate change, whether it is domestic or foreign (Stern, 2007). New technologies, for example, hydraulic fracturing, make untapped sources of energy more accessible, but the environmental cost is high with water pollution and earthquakes (Manuel, 2010; Howarth et al., 2011). Greenhouse gas concentrations are increasing at alarming rates from usage of petroleum products (Stern, 2007). The public debate about whether this is causing climate change is amazing to scientists because the data does not lie. Clearly these molecules in the air are trapping infrared rays and not allowing re-radiation of heat back into space (Samimi and Zarinabadi, 2012). This effect of petroleum is a strong argument for moving to bio-based fuels, energy, and products to slow climate change and provide renewable, degradable products.

The world population is growing exponentially and will reach 10 billion by the year 2050 (Altman and Hasegawa, 2012). These people increase the demand for food and energy—the individual desire for food, particularly meat, and energy will increase with an increase in socioeconomic status in developing countries. Thus, a 50% increase in food production is required just to meet the status quo for an increase in the number of people living on the planet. However, because of the increasing demand for meat, the current calories produced will not suffice, because when primary plant productivity flows through an animal in the food chain, only 10% of that primary productivity is transferrable through meat to humans.

In the United States, the public does not understand food production. Food-related jobs for all areas of processing involve less than 5% of the population (private research question answered by K. Hood in a personal communication, Bureau of Economic Analysis), and the planting and care of crops as well as harvesting occur with less than 2% of the US population (http://data.worldbank.org/indicator/SL.AGR.EMPL.ZS). The boxes of cereal and loaves of bread along with fresh or frozen fruits and vegetables are available any time of the year. Farmers use tractors to plow soils to prepare them for planting in order to plant seeds, cultivate, and harvest, using fossil fuels for each action. In addition, fertilizers, herbicides, insecticides, and fungicides are added to the crops to protect them from nutrient starvation, weeds, insects, and diseases. Each of these actions requires fossil fuels for application, and the chemicals are often also made using fossil fuel feedstock.

In spite of the fact that agriculture is not understood, in many circles it is considered a sacred concept. Small farmers and family farms suggest an aura of pastoral tranquility and communing with nature. Most farmers do what they can to protect their land and thus their livelihood. However, they farm to make money, and making money demands inputs for high yields. Indeed, the harvests are impressive in US agriculture, but the practices are on borrowed time. Inputs comprise large amounts of water in addition to the chemicals listed above. Since the 1970s, and the advent of the Green Revolution, breeding, fertilizer, and irrigation have been used to increase productivity on a worldwide scale (Jain, 2010). These are the tools that have been available to agricultural scientists. However, we are now in need of increasing productivity without increasing inputs, and sometimes even lowering inputs such as water and fertilizer. These agricultural crop productivity improvements are important for biofuels and bio-based product production as well as for food and feed.

Potential Solutions: Technologies

New technologies such as synthetic biology, biotechnology, genomics, transcriptomics, and proteomics have revolutionized the way science is conducted and the speed with which new information is obtained. The problem with these new technologies is that they are complex and not understandable to the general public. Thus, it generates distrust in the process no matter what the results. However, if one considers the explosion in electronic technologies and their adoption by the public, it is clear that not all technologies are met with the same distrust. How many users of data phones and personal computers understand those technologies?

What are these new scientific tools, and how do they work? Biotechnology may be the most familiar because it has been around for approximately 40 years. Biotechnology, in this case, involves molecular cloning of genes, which are composed of DNA, the genetic material of life. Molecular cloning is the production of multiple copies of a piece of DNA. The first genes were cloned during the 1970s by Boyer et al. (Cohen et al., 1973). The clone was a joining of two plasmids, small circular pieces of DNA from *Escherichia coli* (*E. coli*), a workhorse organism in the laboratory. These joined pieces of DNA (Fig. 8.1) were put back into *E. coli*. Numerous animal genes were later spliced into these self-replicating plasmids in order to study the function of these genes and their protein products.

This molecular cloning, or molecular biotechnology, generates genetically engineered organisms. The technology is very precise and allows changes in an organism's productivity or other characteristics (Handa et al., 2012; Lers, 2012; Samach, 2012; Topp and Benfey, 2012). The potential traits that can be

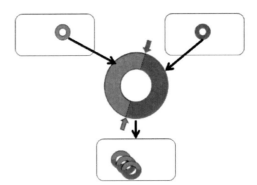

Figure 8.1 A new plasmid is created from the joining of two plasmids. After introduction into a new *E. coli* cell, multiple identical copies of the new plasmid are formed, creating a molecular cloning event.

engineered for increasing plant productivity are vast. However, to determine the best genes and traits to use will require good hypotheses and lots of experimentation with knowledge gained through other new technologies.

Other new technologies comprise the "omics" technologies. The first of these to be developed was genomics, or the ability to know the entire sequence of all the genes of an organism. The human genome (DNA) sequence was the first whole sequence known (Venter et al., 2001). Subsequent to the human genome sequence, a model plant genome, *Arabidopsis*, and several key crop plant genomes were sequenced, for example, maize (Arabidopsis, 2000; Schnable et al., 2009). Although the DNA sequence itself is very interesting, the greater utility of the genome sequence is to understand how a plant becomes a plant or an animal becomes an animal.

The central dogma of biology is how the DNA, or genes, becomes proteins that can do work in a microbe, plant, or animal (Fig. 8.2). The cellular machinery copies a strand of the DNA (the gene) into a message, and the message is then translated into a protein. The central dogma illustrates two other levels of investigation to understand life, the message (transcripts of the genes) and the proteins. One can measure the messenger RNA

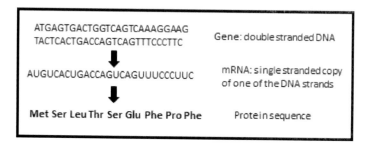

Figure 8.2 The central dogma of biology. Double-stranded DNA is copied into messenger RNA (mRNA). In this case it is copied from the lower strand and matches the top DNA strand. mRNA has uracil (U) in place of thymine (T). Each set of three bases encodes one amino acid. The protein in the third line is encoded from the mRNA.

(mRNA) (the transcriptome) and the proteins (the proteome). The mRNA molecules vary in number and reflect how much each gene is working to create life in any particular cell or tissue at a particular time. The mRNAs can be sequenced, counted, and matched to the DNA genome sequence so that we can understand changes or variations that display the final visual and chemical characteristics of the plant or animal. The complete set of proteins of an organism's cells or tissues can also be determined. The interactions of these "omics" technologies have taken us far into the story of life but, to date, not the entire story. We still have much to learn about how life works.

New plant, animal, and microbial varieties can be generated using these tools. However, manipulating gene sets to improve traits is possible only after we figure out how these organisms work. We must use all the technological tools discussed above to achieve the pressing productivity goals. Even the creator of the Green Revolution, Dr. Norman Bourlag, advocated moving to biotechnology and genomics to continue creating improvements in plant productivity for agriculture saying, "If the naysayers do manage to stop agricultural biotechnology, they might actually precipitate the famines and the crisis of global biodiversity they have been predicting for nearly 40 years" (http://www.hoover.org/publications/defining-ideas/article/108641).

Product Example Using Technologies

Plants and microbes have been used for hundreds of years to produce molecules of importance to industry and medicine. In most early cases, these were natural products from the metabolism of organisms. With the advent of biotechnology, however, more products can now be made in these organisms, often in higher amounts, allowing enzymes, medicines, and vaccines to be produced in abundance and at low cost. An example of this is the production of an industrial enzyme in corn kernels using biotechnology and transcriptomics.

RB	Promoter	Gene of Interest	Terminator	S	Selection Cassette	LB

Figure 8.3 The general structure of a gene insertion cassette into a plant. Our gene of interest can be from any source: plant, animal, or microbial. However, it must have regulatory sequences such as a promoter and a terminator that tell the gene how to be expressed in the plant. The promoter and terminator are most often from plant origin, although they can also be derived from plant viruses or bacterial symbionts. The selection cassette represents a gene that can be used to identify plant cells that have received the linked gene of interest. The selection can be antibiotic or herbicide resistance, among others. S = spacer DNA; RB = right border of *Agrobacterium tumefaciens* (*A. tumefaciens*) transferred DNA (T-DNA); LB = left border of *A. tumefaciens* T-DNA.

The process of plant biotechnology takes genes from any source and puts them into a plant to produce new proteins of interest. Whenever this occurs, one must also include plant sequences that tell the plant when and where to produce the new proteins. These sequences include the promoter, which tells the plant when and where to transcribe the genes into mRNA, and the terminator, which tells the plant when to stop the transcription of mRNA. The gene insertion cassettes are put together in *E. coli* using molecular biotechnology and then put into a vector with a right border (RB) and a left border (LB) that define the length of the cassettes (Fig. 8.3). Then the genes are moved into plant cells.

Figure 8.4 illustrates the process of moving the gene from the vector into the plant chromosomes. We use a natural process that

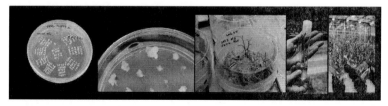

Figure 8.4 The process of corn transformation and regeneration. From embryo culture in panel 1 through seed harvest in panel 5 usually takes from 9 to 12 months.

harnesses the magic of *A. tumefaciens* to move the gene from the vector into the plant chromosomes. We start with immature corn embryos that are cocultured with the bacterial strain that contains our gene of interest, as shown in Fig. 8.3. Once the gene is inserted into a chromosome within a single cell, this cell can be encouraged to grow and produce more cells on a medium that contains an herbicide or other selective chemical (panel 2). These cells are then induced to form embryos that will germinate into a small plantlet (panel 3), which after rooting (panel 4) can be planted in the greenhouse. The whole plant regenerated from that single cell contains the gene of interest in every cell of the new plant. This means that the plant can produce seeds that also contain the gene and the protein.

Our process uses this agricultural biotechnology to produce enzymes (catalytic proteins) in a plant seed. The seed itself is a biofactory for these enzymes rather than fungal cultures in large fermenter tanks. Our product, the enzyme cellulase, can economically convert cellulose, the principle component of plant bodies, into sugars that can be made into biofuels. The market for these cellulase products is projected by 2022 to be at least $0.5 billion.

One of the enzymes that can partially degrade cellulose is an endocellulase called E1. We took a gene for this endocellulase from a thermostable bacterium, *Acidothermus cellulolyticus*, which was found growing in a hot spring in Yellowstone National Park. The gene was cloned using molecular biotechnology (described above) into an *E. coli* vector first and then combined with plant sequences so that the gene could be recognized by the plant and would make the enzyme. Figure 8.3 shows the structure of the plant-related gene sequences for the enzyme that was transferred into the plant. Figure 8.4 illustrates how the gene is moved into the corn plant. This process generates many plants containing the gene.

Once we have the seed, we can determine how much protein is present in the seed and choose the best plants to use for product development. The enzymes can be purified or formulated as concentrated extracts of seeds and sold into different applications such as research for biomass conversion or pulp processing for paper manufacture. The advantage of using plants for making the enzymes is that they are a renewable resource and require very little capital infrastructure, that is, steel in the ground. For large product volume demands, this is critical. Planting more acreage can increase plant-made enzymes instead of building more vats to grow fungal-based enzymes.

We have taken the production lines and looked at them with transcriptomics technology to understand why some corn lines produce high amounts of the recombinant (transgenic) protein and others do not. Thus we are utilizing some of the cutting-edge technologies to try to make the maximum product for the least expense. The results of transcriptomics should help us choose the best production lines at an early stage, allowing rural economic development as well energy independence for renewable products from plants.

Conclusions

Traditionally, agricultural research and technology transfer have been grossly underfunded. If this research had been funded at a level similar to medical research, we might have met some of these goals that are so urgent and apparent now. The United States needs to consider the consequences of underfunding agricultural research in the 21st century because of the demands for food/feed/fiber and fuel for present and future generations.

Current food production in the United States allows for quite inexpensive prices. Unfortunately, the prices are supported by government subsidies and do not reflect the actual prices of production. This is fortunate for the working poor but is not necessary for middle- and upper-class families. Food and energy prices are quite low compared to those in the rest of the world. This allows overconsumption and waste, while other cultures are suffering from lack of supply.

The utility of new tools for plant productivity improvements is amazing. Biotechnology as well as "omics" technologies can be utilized to improve disease and insect resistance, nitrogen use efficiency, and water use efficiency for improved production. In addition, these improvements can be applied to crops that are being targeted for pharmaceutical or industrial applications so that the utilization of green plants does not detract from food and feed needs. Future research needs to be funded at the highest levels to improve our ability to grow the necessary biomass to feed and clothe the world's increasing population, as well as to supply industrial products.

References

Altman, A., and Hasegawa, P. M. (2012). *Plant Biotechnology and Agriculture: Prospects for the 21st Century*. London: Academic Press.

Arabidopsis, G. I. (2000). Analysis of the genome sequence of the flowering plant Arabidopsis thaliana. *Nature*, **408**(6814), 796.

Cohen, S. N., Chang, A. C., Boyer, H. W., and Helling, R. B. (1973). Construction of biologically functional bacterial plasmids in vitro. *Proceedings of the National Academy of Sciences of the United States of America*, **70**(11), 3240–3244.

Handa, A. K., Tiznado-Hernandez, M.-E., and Mattoo, A. K. (2012). Fruit development and ripening: a molecular perspective, in *Plant Biotechnology and Agriculture: Prospects for the 21st Century*, Altman, A., and Hasegawa, P. M. (eds.), 405–424. London: Academic Press.

Howarth, R. W., Ingraffea, A., and Engelder, T. (2011). Natural gas: should fracking stop? *Nature*, **477**(7364), 271–275.

Jain, H. K. (2010). *The Green Revolution: History, Impact and Future*. Houston, TX: Studium Press.

Lers, A. (2012). Potential application of biotechnology to maintain fresh produce postharvest quality and reduce losses during storage, in *Plant Biotechnology and Agriculture: Prospects for the 21st Century*, Altman, A., and Hasegawa, P. M. (eds.), 425–442. London: Academic Press.

Manuel, J. (2010). EPA tackles fracking. *Environmental Health Perspectives*, **118**(5), A199.

Rosin, H. (2013). The touch-screen generation: young children—even toddlers—are spending more and more time with digital technology. What will it mean for their development? *The Atlantic*, **2013/04**, 1–12.

Samach, A. (2012). Control of flowering, in *Plant Biotechnology and Agriculture: Prospects for the 21st Century*, Altman, A., and Hasegawa, P. M. (eds.), 387–404. London: Academic Press.

Samimi, A., and Zarinabadi, S. (2012). Reduction of greenhouse gases emission and effect on environment. *Journal of American Science*, **8**(8), 1011–1015.

Schnable, P. S., Ware, D., Fulton, R. S., Stein, J. C., Wei, F., Pasternak, S., . . . and Wilson, R. K. (2009). The B73 maize genome: complexity, diversity, and dynamics. *Science*, **326**, 1112–1115.

Stern, N. (2007). *The Economics of Climate Change: The Stern Review*. Cambridge, UK: Cambridge University Press.

Topp, C. N., and Benfey, P. N. (2012). Growth control of root architecture, in *Plant Biotechnology and Agriculture: Prospects for the 21st Century*, Altman, A., and Hasegawa, P. M. (eds.), 373–386. London: Academic Press, Elsevier.

Venter, J. C., Adams, M. D., Myers, E. W., Li, P. W., Mural, R. J., Sutton, G. G., . . . and Zhu, X. (2001). The sequence of the human genome. *Science Signaling*, **291**(5507), 1304.

Soon They'll Know Our Secrets

Rosalyn W. Berne

A species smaller than the eye can see
Or larger than most living things
And yet we take from it without consent
Our shelter, food, habiliment
　　　　　　　　　　　　—Stevie Wonder

WITH PREDAWN THE MOISTURE grew heavy, falling as droplets across the leaves of the trees and settling as dew on the grasses. Soon the sun's rays would remove the sweet wetness, and the shimmering leaves would exhale.

"What did she say just now?" asked the ancient one, who stood tall outside the concealed windows of the Northern California lab.

"She said, 'Isn't that interesting,'" returned the one whose cells lay broken beneath the eyes of the scope. "She said it as if she now understands."

"That means she's almost unlocked our code," the stately redwood stand cried out, nearly in unison. "Who knows what THEY will do with *that* knowledge!"

"Clearly, the time has come. WE must transmit a message out across the kingdom to determine what may soon need to be done."

"What shall WE say?" the young ones replied, their needles tender and light and newly alive.

The ancient ones pondered. They sent beacons up and down the coast through the Fir, the Maple, and the Birch, which, in turn, spread the signals to the Dogwood, the Willow, the

Redbud, and the Cypress. In response, the Aspen, intertwined as ONE, sent the beacon over the mountains, until the woodlands of the Midwest, the grasses of the plains, the reeds of the lakes and marshes, and all species on the continent had heard the crestfallen cry. The great oak sang out in glory, their vibrations crossing the seas, asking others to contribute to the crucial message. Soon the Redwood inquiry had circumnavigated the globe, and the answer was returned: "WE shall recount the history of the humans, in THEIR relationship with WE. History will teach us what must be *done*."

Dr. Clarissa Mendelssohn worked late in the laboratory, long after her colleagues left for home. She was too close to stop, feeling more intrigue than fatigue as she suppressed her excitement. It was too soon for celebration, or self-pride. Something could still go wrong. DNA extraction from plant tissues, unlike DNA isolation from mammalian tissues, had been difficult to achieve. The rigid walls around the plant's cells made it a daunting endeavor. Laborious mechanical grinding had been required to disrupt the cell wall, thus releasing the DNA, only to provide incomplete and sparse information.

Eventually, using carbohydrases enabled complete digestion of plant cell walls and subsequent DNA release. It continued to be a very long process to extract the resulting simple sugars and the high-yield, high-molecular weight DNA. Humans have acquired detailed DNA sequences for few classified plant species, most having DNA sequences for only a few genes. But now, through the meticulous work of Dr. Mendelssohn, push-button sequencing and assembly of all of earth's complex plant genomes would finally be achieved.

She'd not published results in over two years, hesitant to share all that she was learning or how quickly her work was coming to completion, until she was absolutely sure. At times she berated herself for her competitiveness, but professional motivations led her to remain stealthy. Whether prideful, curious, self-doubting, or elated, her feelings were received directly by the ancient ones, whose trunks stood outside her windows and whose roots extended beneath her laboratory. Dr. Mendelssohn's head swooned with the possibilities of having access to the complete genomes of the entire plant kingdom.

Tonight, it seemed, or perhaps by morning, the full sequencing of the half million plant species alive on earth would finally be complete. Who would ever believe her? What would happen then? Many others were seeking to achieve the very same, knowing it would mean that the entire plant world, not just a few thousand species, could be put to work as a grand machine, to provide the energy, the medicine, and even the water that humans now most desperately needed. Clarissa thought about this as she worked, and the Redwood responded with a shudder.

"WE shall begin at the beginning," the most ancient one said, its thousand-year branches embracing all the life around it. "WE must remember back to the first days." The discreet messages began to form into a collective sense within the kingdom. The vibrational transmission to all began early in the middle of the night:

> *WE emerged to support their lives on earth, over the course of millions and millions of years. WE evolved until finally the land was ready for them. They climbed out of the sea, and all of existence was perfectly in balance: healthy, strong, and supportive of their evolution as hominids. When they stood up and began to carry tools it was necessary for WE to adjust, to maintain our tender connection with they. But they soon lost their sense of the connection with WE, and decreed domination and control.*
>
> *Even still, WE continued with they and complied, to ensure their bellies and lungs would be filled and that their exhaled wastes would be absorbed. WE extended our seeds, fruits, stems, roots, and leaves for ingestion so that their blood would be strong and well*

nourished. WE offered our trunks and limbs for their shelter and for their transportation across the lands and the sea. Despite the widening gap between us, WE continued to fulfill our purpose: WE were to support the lives of they who were here to keep God from being lonely.

Clarissa removed the final plant sample and added more of its cells to her diffusion. Returning it to the flow cytometer instrument she'd redesigned and had built, the only one of its kind in the world, she sat quietly on the stool at her bench, waiting patiently as the lasers did their work. Her laboratory, also a greenhouse, held thousands of species of plant life that no person had yet completely sequenced. Clarissa's one slight alteration in the machine had accelerated the process a thousand-fold.

The last of her collection, the rare plant *Philcoxia minensis*, was discovered growing in the tropical savannas of Brazil. Such an unusual specimen—some of the plant's millimeter-wide leaves grow above ground, but most of its tiny, sticky leaves burrow beneath the surface of the white sands. "Why would evolution do that?" is the question that haunted Clarissa, one she asked the plant directly as she prepared it for final analysis. The worm-digesting carnivore would soon have no choice but to reveal its secrets to humanity.

"Hello there," she mumbled to herself, though her tone was as if the plant might actually hear and understand.

"We know the effects of drought on plants. We understand how you obtain nutrients from the soil. Everyone knows that plants react to light, that plants use volatile chemicals to communicate with each other. But did your perception of sound and vibrations evolve, too? And can you sense me speaking to you?"

Philcoxia did, indeed, sense Clarissa; only she did not, in turn, sense its response.

Perhaps it was the fatigue that drew this strange talking from Clarissa. That is what she began to suspect as night edged toward morning. The plants felt her anxiety as well as her exhaustion. Meanwhile, the transmission continued:

> *THEIR practices became increasingly destructive, with entire forests decimated into farms, ranches, and cities, making it more and more difficult for WE to breathe. The more they cut, the less water there was in the aquifers, in the soil, in the rivers, and in the atmosphere of the earth. The roots of WE felt more and more stressed in search of the nutrients needed to thrive. But still, adjustments were made, and WE adapted as best as WE could. Continuing to support their well-being was imperative, though their dominion had become capricious and wanton. The existence of WE would soon be threatened.*

Clarissa took a leaf, a stem, and a piece of root, placing them into a centrifuge to create the solution. Then she deposited its sludge, the final step of her method, into the core of her instrument for analysis. Peering into the scope she observed the process as the genes were individually dissected. The screen above her revealed the intricate pattern of the plant's unique life. A feeling of awe swelled in her breast, and her eyes welled up in fearful joy. The plants in her lab, and the shrubs, bulbs, bushes, and trees outside, all sensed her elation. For all these years of her research endeavors WE had and sought to support the inquiries of her mind and the compassion of her heart. From then on, however, WE's involvement would entirely depend on her next steps.

"Soon. Very soon now," the ancient ones said to one another. "The last piece of the intricate puzzle will be in place, and WE will be completely revealed to her."

WE had come to love the humans with great tenderness and care. But human knowledge had progressed past human wisdom, putting the kingdom into severe jeopardy. For WE, human life was to be protected at all costs. Except that WE could not provide for the humans if WE itself did not flourish. There were few remaining strategies for survival.

Clarissa ended her long day's work with a sense of tremendous accomplishment. The only thing left to do was to recount her exact methodology in detail and to document the codes in their totality. It would take many weeks to draft the paper for submission to journals for publication. But an informal announcement to the scientific world could be made immediately:

> "The complete genome of the entire plant kingdom has now been mapped," is all it said.

Clarissa stepped out of the lab into the first rays of morning, her eyes squinting in response to the brightness. As she walked through the grove of tall trees, WE felt and absorbed the vibrations of her passing. WE knew what she had done.

The boulevard was already busy with the onset of rush hour as she pulled out of the parking lot and onto the entry ramp. Concrete lay before and behind her, and concrete buildings rose above, the glass windows displaying the reflected sky. Planes crisscrossed white trails in the atmosphere, as the sounds of the city created a cacophony. Once home, Clarissa got the well-deserved sleep she needed. Except for the disturbance of the dream . . .

She dreamed she was laying on a sticky surface. All around her were the deep green leaves of a single plant, curling inward and covering her body. At first she had the sensation of being cradled, cared for in a mothering way. Then the horror emerged. She realized she was unable to turn or move in any way. Locked into immobility she tried with all her might to scream. But she was unable to open her mouth. And then she heard the murmur, a subtle vibration at first, then more energized. She moaned with trepidation. She could feel it coursing through her limbs. Was it speaking to her?

WE waited as long as possible, adapting and evolving as they learned and grew in the capacity to recreate life. WE hesitated, intending to continue our service. It pains WE that this is what WE must now do.

As the leaves closed tightly around Clarissa, and the digestive enzymes began to flow into her pores, the sound of her own screaming voice awakened her.

"Only a dream," she reassured herself. Greatly relieved she fell back asleep. And the kingdom of WE awakened as ONE to activate the only choice it had left.

Chapter 9

The Promise and Pitfalls of Cognitive Enhancement

David Carmel

Psychology Department, University of Edinburgh, 7 George Square, Edinburgh EH8 9JZ, UK

dave.carmel@ed.ac.uk

> To light a candle is to cast a shadow.
> —Ursula K. Le Guin, *A Wizard of Earthsea*

You might be familiar with what I'm going through: As I sit down to write this essay, I am finding it very hard to just get on with it. Endless distractions—e-mails, phone calls, yesterday's leftovers in the fridge—interfere with my concentration; the many aspects of the topic I want to write about keep getting garbled in my mind, leading me to forget details and curtailing the creation of a logical, ordered formulation of ideas; and I find myself wishing I could do something else—maybe go for a walk or watch a movie—and get back to this later. Wouldn't it be great if there were something I could do to increase my focus, boost my memory, and improve my motivation, something effortless like taking a pill to give me the mental charge I lack right now?

Creating Life from Life: Biotechnology and Science Fiction
Edited by Rosalyn W. Berne
Copyright © 2015 Pan Stanford Publishing Pte. Ltd.
ISBN 978-981-4463-58-4 (Hardcover), 978-981-4463-59-1 (eBook)
www.panstanford.com

There may be. Recent years have seen a significant increase in the nonclinical use of drugs that are usually prescribed for other purposes, but are used "off label" to boost various aspects of cognition—so-called "smart drugs." Most users of such drugs have never been diagnosed with attention deficit or any other disorder (neither have I) and function well within the norm. It is also within the norm, however, to feel that the challenges we encounter in the course of a busy, modern-day life—the constant demand to do *better*, passing exams and completing projects on tight schedules—tax our brains to a point we are barely able to handle. Smart drugs may represent a potential solution.

The use of drugs to enhance human cognitive function is one of the most contentious issues in modern neuroscience (Farah, Parens, Sahakian, and Wolpe, 2004; Frenguelli, 2013): Can we really enhance cognitive performance by pharmacological means? And perhaps more importantly, *should* we? I am a psychologist, not a pharmacologist, so I won't focus here on the first of these questions. I am interested in the second one—to what extent is pharmacological cognitive enhancement desirable? How will it affect the way individuals function and feel about themselves, and what will a society in which smart drugs are prevalent be like?

The Candle

Let's start with the current state of affairs. How widespread is the use of pharmacological cognitive enhancement? The estimates obtained from surveys vary widely: Amongst students in the United States, the reported use of prescription drugs to improve concentration and memory while studying ranges from 5% to 35% (Smith and Farah, 2011). A poll of 1400 academic scientists conducted by *Nature* magazine a few years ago (Maher, 2008) found that about 20% of them had used cognitive enhancers for nonmedical purposes (a further 15% had them prescribed for medical reasons).

The numbers suggest that even if the use of smart drugs is not yet the norm, it is nonetheless a significant trend. But surveys are notoriously unreliable—the samples may not be representative (Ragan, Bard, and Singh, 2013), and the phrasing of survey questions may be ambiguous or conflate medical, off-label, and recreational uses (Schleim, 2010). Furthermore, people might not answer truthfully (e.g., because they used illegal means such as online sources to obtain the drugs; the dangers of using unreliable suppliers are significant but not directly relevant to the present topic). We therefore need better estimates of how prevalent the use of prescription drugs for cognitive enhancement really is (Nadler and Reiner, 2010).

The prescription drugs that have been appropriated for cognitive enhancement are, for the most part, medications that were developed to treat psychiatric and neurological disorders but may also improve performance in similar domains in healthy people (Greely et al., 2008). The most commonly used are Ritalin (the commercial name of methylphenidate) and Adderall (mixed amphetamine salts), which are usually prescribed for the treatment of attention deficit hyperactivity disorder (ADHD) but are used off label to boost attention and concentration; Provigil (modafinil), which is prescribed for fatigue and narcolepsy but is also being used to maintain alertness and wakefulness; and Aricept (donepezil), which was developed to treat Alzheimer's disease but is being used to enhance memory.

Surprisingly, in light of the hype these drugs have received, the jury is still out on whether they really do improve cognitive function and, if so, to what extent. While there is some evidence for the effectiveness of the above medications in off-label usage, the evidence for specific cognitive enhancement in healthy populations is weak and requires further validation. In the research conducted so far, the results have been inconsistent and the effect sizes small (Ragan et al., 2013).

Furthermore, it is important to understand that even if such drugs did show strong cognitive enhancement effects, this would still not be enough to sanction such use: These drugs operate by a host of chemical mechanisms, not all of which are fully understood. A drug that affects a chemical pathway in a part of the brain that is involved in memory, for example, will also affect the same chemical pathway—and perhaps other chemical pathways, too—in other parts of the nervous system. The side effects of drugs are often unpredictable (those of modafinil, for example, include skin rashes, depression, and heart problems), and risking them may not be justified outside the context of treating an even-worse medical condition. The potential for a drug to be addictive must also be ruled out before it can be doled out for nonmedical purposes. We're not there yet.

The Light

Let's imagine a future in which the teething problems of pharmacological cognitive enhancement have been overcome. It's never easy to predict the timing of such future developments, but in light of the massive potential market for smart drugs and the fact that both academic scientists and commercial drug manufacturers are putting considerable effort into developing them, it seems reasonable to assume this future may not be too far off.

So imagine that cognitive enhancement really works—the next generation of smart drugs reliably improves concentration, memory, alertness, and motivation. In our speculative-but-just-around-the-corner future, these drugs specifically target the neural systems that underlie the abilities they enhance: a memory-enhancing drug does not affect the many other parts of the brain and nervous system that use the same chemical pathways. These drugs are thus free of side effects. Furthermore, they can be purchased from trustworthy legitimate sources, are not physiologically addictive, work for nearly everyone who takes them, and can be taken whenever and for however long they are needed. For the purpose of this exercise, in other words, let's imagine an extreme situation that will allow us to explore the full implications for a world that has ideal cognitive enhancement drugs. I won't bother with regulatory issues such as whether these drugs will require a prescription; people have a way of getting their hands on things that are important enough to them, and our main concern here is the effects that the very existence of such drugs might have on people's lives, rather than how their administration will be managed.

Effective cognitive enhancement has the power to transform many aspects of the way we live, and do so rapidly: Think how the Internet has completely changed the way we conduct many of our affairs, in just a couple of decades. The changes brought about by widely available cognitive enhancement may be more subtle—they might not alter the outside appearance of the way people study and work—but also more profound, ultimately dwarfing the online revolution.

Our world is dominated by the need for people do to cognitively demanding work. To function successfully in most educational and work environments, one must continuously process and remember information and keep doing so for prolonged periods. If smart drugs had somehow become available a few hundred years ago, when most people were farmers and manual laborers, they may not have made much of a difference; nowadays, in a world of surgeons, pilots, stockbrokers, attorneys, computer programmers, and air-traffic controllers (and of course, students of all these and other professions) it might be hard to overestimate the magnitude of the difference such drugs will make.

Perhaps the most obvious implications have to do with competence, at both individual and societal levels. As individuals, we will all be able to do better—to concentrate for longer, retain more information, use this information effectively, and do so for longer at a time. We will not have to worry about forgetting an important fact during a presentation or losing our train of thought during a job interview; we will be able to find our focus and meet deadlines without the stress that accompanies distraction. Different drugs will have different effects—some may impact those who must be productive, improving their ability to complete tasks such as writing articles or computer code. Others will affect those who have jobs where one needs to be alert, constantly making sure that airplanes don't crash into each other or that no one in the pool is drowning. Certain professions may enjoy both types of benefits, such as when radiologists need to apply their expertise to decipher large numbers of magnetic resonance imaging (MRI) scans in search of tumors.

The potential benefits are definitely not limited to the kind of high-end, skilled work that requires a substantial education. Take baggage screening personnel at airports, for example— those people who have to look at an endless stream of X-rays of suitcases going by on a conveyor belt, monitoring them carefully because there is a minuscule chance that one of them might contain a bomb, a weapon, or an illicit substance. This might be one of the most tedious jobs on earth, but it requires relentless alertness and concentration. Research has shown that when people, even highly accomplished specialists, need to search for something visually, they are more likely to miss their target if it is unexpected (Drew, Vo, and Wolfe, 2012) or rare (Evans, Evered, Tambouret, Wilbur, and Wolfe, 2011; Wolfe, Horowitz, and Kenner, 2005). In a set of equally complex displays (e.g., suitcases that are all roughly the same size and contain a similar number of items), a target such as a gun is less likely to be spotted if it is present in 1 out of every 10,000 displays than if it is present in 1 out of 100. The problem is that in reality, suitcases containing guns and bombs and the like are exceedingly rare. People, even dedicated security workers, get bored; with such odds, even the most conscientious and motivated begin to slack off. There are various ways to improve performance—managers might arrange shorter shifts or artificially plant suitcases containing target items to make them more common and increase the chances they will be discovered. But a pharmacological intervention that made it possible for people to remain focused on a repetitive, monotonous task so that they would hardly ever miss a dangerous target—that would be a huge step forward. It would, quite literally, make the world a safer place.

The technological advancements of the modern world have allowed automation to take many of the more tedious aspects of work out of human hands. It may be a while before we trust our technology to handle airport baggage screening with little or no human oversight, but many other jobs are now left in the capable hands of machines and computers. Humans cannot be taken out of the loop completely, though: a person still has to get involved whenever something goes wrong or when anything unexpected, which wasn't explicitly programmed into the machinery, happens. And in such cases, the human action usually needs to be swift, decisive, and most importantly, competent.

Airliners are nowadays flown almost entirely (except for short periods during takeoff and landing) by a computerized autopilot; but an autopilot cannot save the day when the plane's engines go bust, by making a bold decision to land in a river. On January 15, 2009, US Airways Captain Chesley Sullenberger did just that—he landed Flight 1549 in the Hudson River, saving the lives of all 155 people on board after a flock of birds had disabled both of his Airbus A320's engines. Sullenberger has become a national hero; the noteworthy aspect of his action, however, was not bravery but competence. It is widely acknowledged that most professional pilots would find it hard to pull off what Sullenberger did, and he himself has attributed his success at the moment of truth to his 42 years of experience. It is precisely in those situations, where our reliance on technology breaks down and competent human action is required, where pharmacological interventions that guarantee professionals' ability to always be at the top of their game may be most important.

If the benefits of reduced human error and increased productivity are applied at a large scale, they will result in a society in which things *work*—better and more reliably than ever before. People will be safer, receive higher quality health care, and accomplish a lot more. Such a society will set an unprecedented standard for what constitutes a job well done; and if we can all do better, we will soon have no excuse not to.

The Shadow

In a world where pharmacological cognitive enhancement is effective and accessible, the benefits of improved cognitive performance will soon come to be taken for granted. Think of the transformation that interpersonal communication has undergone since the advent of cell phones: we now expect people to be reachable at any time, and tend to get annoyed if they don't answer their phone or at least get back to us quickly (and "quickly" has itself been truncated from "sometime today" to "it's been half an hour; how dare he?"). In a similar vein, once the level of performance engendered by cognitive enhancement becomes the norm, prepharmacological performance levels will become unacceptable.

In various lines of work—most notably, those in which constant top-notch performance is a safety or profitability requirement—the use of cognitive enhancers will probably go beyond being a norm to becoming compulsory. This may affect not only pilots and surgeons, whose mistakes could cost lives, but even stockbrokers, whose errors cost their employers money. The level of informed consent available to employees in this scenario raises serious concerns about the amount of free choice they will have (Hyman, Volkow, and Nutt, 2013). In fact, employers might not have much of a choice about whether to make cognitive enhancement mandatory—it is likely to be a basic condition of insurance policies.

In education, the use of cognitive enhancers will change from something students do to get ahead into a minimal requirement for not falling behind. Students who want to get by on their own raw intellect, however powerful, may find themselves at a disadvantage. The difference between students who do and don't use cognitive enhancers may be so clear, and not using enhancers may be so off the table as an option, that the use of enhancers might become not only sanctioned but even mandated by educational institutions—if you're training someone to be a doctor, you want them to already be the best they can possibly be during training, right?

All the above might not sound so bad—after all, society as a whole will reap the rewards of competence detailed in the previous section. But such developments will not come without costs and some novel dilemmas.

Pharmacological cognitive enhancement opens up a whole new dimension for peer pressure and competition between individuals (Scheske and Schnall, 2012). Even ubiquitous and accessible cognitive enhancers are likely to be costly, opening a new type of divide between the haves and have-nots: where once a student from a poor background might have been able to overcome his or her disadvantaged starting point through talent and hard work, the bar set by peers who enjoy a chemical boost may be too high to overcome by natural means. And even if the smart drugs at our disposal are as ideal as I postulated earlier—targeting specific neural systems with no side effects—everybody is a little different, and there will always be those whose physiological and genetic makeup make them less susceptible to the effects of such drugs, reducing the benefits they may get from them; and of course, there will always be those—perhaps very few—who are allergic. Some children, then, will be left behind, not for lack of aptitude and effort, but simply because of the chemical makeup of their bodies.

Economic considerations may also affect the decision to use cognitive enhancers at an institutional level. The difference between schools that can supply their students with enhancers and those that cannot may open the door to a whole new, two-tiered education system. The struggle to get in, keep up, and get ahead has been in place for generations—but it may take less than one generation for it to become drug dependent.

This drug dependence is perhaps the key dilemma we will face: We will have to choose the extent to which we want to live in a society where anything that can be evaluated—and this includes an ever-expanding sphere of domains—requires the consumption of pharmacological substances if it is to run in a way that is deemed acceptable. This choice will be made at both regulatory/legal and cultural levels, and there is likely to be a tension between the legal stipulations and cultural norms that evolve.

All this, some will say, is just whiny fear of progress. Every advancement in history has been challenged by those who saw it as unnatural or as a threat to social order. According to this view, smart drugs are not like cocaine but like reading glasses: Yes, they are artificial, but they give people the ability to do things they couldn't do without them. Not everyone will be able to use them, but that's just the price you pay for introducing something new that makes the world a better place.

Whether the world at large will indeed be a better place is open to debate, as I described above. As a psychologist, however, my main interest is how cognitive enhancement might affect the individuals who use it. The comparison with glasses is a good opportunity to ask, are smart drugs really just the same as having a new instrument that can help you see better?

To me, there seems to be a clear difference. Glasses are a tool, whereas cognitive enhancers change something about who and what you are. This opinion is a gut feeling; I could probably construct a full, rational argument for it, but I am aware that gut feelings are a product of culture and personal history. Once cognitive enhancers become commonplace, people's intuitions about whether they differ qualitatively from glasses might change.

I am concerned, however, about the relationship people will have with their own achievements. Think of your accomplishments, the ones you are most proud of, those that required that you demonstrate skill, perseverance, and talent.

Now imagine that you had achieved those accomplishments under the influence of smart drugs. Would you still feel as responsible for what you have done as you do now? Many of us base a substantial portion of our self-esteem on our accomplishments in life. What would become of this self-esteem if those accomplishments could be attributed to the effects of drugs that altered the natural workings of our brain? And what about our loved ones, the people we want to be proud of? Would you be as proud of your daughter when she graduated at the top of her college class if you knew this would not have happened without the aid of pharmacological agents?

Human beings are inherently motivated by a need for achievement—the desire to work hard toward the attainment of difficult goals and be recognized for having done so. This need has long been considered a fundamental aspect of personality (Murray, 1938). People may differ in how dominant the need for achievement is for them; for some, other needs may be stronger—these include the desire to build strong social bonds (need for affiliation) and wanting to have strong influence over others (need for power; McClelland, 1961). But we all want to have ownership of our achievements, and this is particularly true for the sorts of people who gravitate toward studies and careers that require hard work and high levels of skill. Now imagine that all those people—doctors, engineers, military officers—perform much better than ever before but cannot fully attribute their successes to their innate abilities or even efforts. Will they be proud of what they accomplish? What will happen to their motivation?

Another relevant concept in this context is self-efficacy—one's belief in one's ability to succeed in specific situations (Bandura, 1977). We tend to develop a sense of self-efficacy gradually as we become better and more experienced at what we do. It is dependent on having accomplished difficult things, endowing us with the belief that we would be able to accomplish them again. The higher our self-efficacy, the more effort we will put into overcoming obstacles. Now, it is certainly possible that someone who is used to performing a difficult, skillful job under the effect of cognitive enhancers would have a healthy sense of self-efficacy; all this requires is that they never need to contemplate the possibility that they might someday be required to perform their job without cognitive enhancement. But is this really how such a person would feel? Would taking smart drugs become such an inherent part of people's self-concept that they would not feel the need to see themselves as capable and competent when they are off the drugs? And even if individuals don't develop a problem with self-efficacy, wouldn't our society as a whole have such a problem—would we not quickly get to a point where the abandonment of cognitive enhancement cannot even be contemplated, as it would sweep the rug from under the foundations that all of society runs on?

I honestly don't know. People are very, very good at coming up with rationalizations, explanations, and excuses. If cognitive enhancement becomes as fundamental as I have been suggesting it might, we may well find a way to explain away the possible undermining of our self-efficacy and need for achievement.

Conclusion

The quote that opens this chapter, from a book by science fiction and fantasy author Ursula K. Le Guin, could apply to any innovation, improvement, or discovery. But the metaphor of a candle seems particularly apt when discussing the human mind: Knowledge itself has always been likened to a flame, and the potential to pharmacologically augment our ability to acquire it leads inevitably to a fundamental change in the way we view our own minds.

It is very likely that before long, we will have to make a choice: As individuals and as a society, do we view pharmacological intervention in the healthy brain's ability to attend to, grasp, and process information as just another one of the ways in which we improve ourselves—alongside getting a good education, eating well, exercising, and wearing glasses? Or do we think of it as a fundamental change in what defines our natural abilities, making pharmacological cognitive enhancement akin to genetically designing babies to have a specific eye color?

These possibilities are the extreme ends of a spectrum of attitudes, with many possible intermediate positions. The specific position we adopt will determine the sort of world we—and I believe it will be us, not our descendants—will find ourselves living in. Personally, I don't think there is a right answer. I wrote this chapter with no boost from any chemicals except caffeine, and have faced anguish caused by lapses in concentration, low motivation in the face of distraction, and the stress of a looming deadline. It would have been great to just be able to sit down, focus for a while, and get it done. A pill that would enable me to do so could make my life so much easier in some ways, but I don't know if I would take it. I am afraid that if I did, I would never again be able to write anything without taking such a pill. The advantages of the candle's light are obvious; but so are the risks that lurk in the shadow.

References

Bandura, A. (1977). Self-efficacy: toward a unifying theory of behavioral change. *Psychological Review*, 84, 191–215.

Drew, T., Vo, M. L.-H., and Wolfe, J. (2012). The invisible gorilla strikes again: sustained attentional blindness in expert observers. *Vision Sciences Society 11th Annual Meeting*.

Evans, K. K., Evered, A., Tambouret, R. H., Wilbur, D. C., and Wolfe, J. M. (2011). Prevalence of abnormalities influences cytologists' error rates in screening for cervical cancer. *Archives of Pathology & Laboratory Medicine*, 135, 1557–1560.

Farah, M. J., Parens, E., Sahakian, B., and Wolpe, P. R. (2004). Neurocognitive enhancement: what can we do and what should we do? *Nature Reviews Neuroscience*, 5, 421–425.

Frenguelli, B. G. (2013). Cognitive enhancers: molecules, mechanisms and minds. *Neuropharmacology*, **64**, 1.

Greely, H., Sahakian, B., Harris, J., Kessler, R. C., Gazzaniga, M., Campbell, P., and Farah, M. J. (2008). Towards responsible use of cognitive-enhancing drugs by the healthy. *Nature*, **456**, 702–705.

Hyman, S., Volkow, N., and Nutt, D. (2013). Pharmacological cognitive enhancement in healthy people: potential and concerns. *Neuropharmacology*, **64**, 8–12.

Maher, B. (2008). Poll results: look who's doping. *Nature*, **452**, 674–675.

McClelland, D. C. (1961). *The Achieving Society*. New York, NY: Free Press.

Murray, H. A. (1938). *Explorations in Personality*. New York, NY: Oxford University Press.

Nadler, R. C., and Reiner, P. B. (2010). A call for data to inform discussion on cognitive enhancement. *BioSocieties*, **5**, 481–487.

Ragan, C. I., Bard, I., and Singh, I. (2013). What should we do about student use of cognitive enhancers? An analysis of current evidence. *Neuropharmacology*, **64**, 588–595.

Scheske, C., and Schnall, S. (2012). The ethics of "smart drugs": moral judgments about healthy people's use of cognitive-enhancing drugs. *Basic and Applied Social Psychology*, **34**, 508–515.

Schleim, S. (2010). Second thoughts on the prevalence of enhancement. *BioSocieties*, **5**, 484–485.

Smith, M. F., and Farah, M. J. (2011). Are prescription stimulants "smart pills"? The epidemiology and cognitive neuroscience of prescription stimulant use by normal healthy individuals. *Psychological Bulletin*, **137**, 717–741.

Wolfe, J. M., Horowitz, T. S., and Kenner, N. (2005). Rare items often missed in visual searches. *Nature*, **435**, 439–440.

Dr. Hyde

David Carmel

I SUPPOSE YOU WANT to know how I did it? How I fooled the biometer?

His tone was challenging but resigned; the discontent in his eyes had nothing to do with the handcuffs or the harsh lighting of the interrogation room. I sat down opposite him.

"Actually, I'm more interested in why."

He lowered his head, revealing a bald patch comically incongruous with his wild sandy hair. His file said he was 33, only 2 years older than me. I continued, "SD-IDs weren't designed for security, you know. They're just there to make sure you have enough Gnosiphen in your blood to start working. Rigging your biochip probably wasn't that hard."

His expression was noncommittal. Better clarify that's not what I'm after. "In any case, it's not my job to figure that out. I'm here to evaluate whether we need to develop SD security now." He looked up. Now he couldn't help looking a tiny bit smug.

"Well, I guess I just proved you do."

"Perhaps. But surely revealing a security breach wasn't what motivated you—you, of all people—to endanger a patient's life?"

"Me of all people?"

"Come on, you know what I'm asking. You're not stupid."

"I'm no brain surgeon either."

So that's where he wanted to go with this. OK. "Ah, but you are. An extraordinary one." His sleeves had been rolled up to make room for the handcuffs, exposing the ID chip implanted in his forearm. Even now, it pulsed with vivid blue-green swirls rather than depleted gray. Looking at it, I added, "SD."

He leaned back in his chair, looking me in the eye, and shrugged. "That's just the State."

I might have to volunteer something here.

"So what?"

He snorted. "It's not . . . Forget it."

No, I couldn't let this slip. "It's not what? Not you?" His shoulders relaxed as he exhaled. Relief?

"That's right."

Good. He actually wanted to talk. But I'd need to supply the sounding board. "You had to have the potential to begin with, though. To be accepted into the program. You know that."

"Is that supposed to make me feel better? That I had potential?"

"No, what you are should do that. State-dependent enhanced cognition means your memory—all the skills you learned, all the judgment—will always be optimal. You're the best you could ever be."

"As long as I'm in State. See, that's what no one realizes till it's too late, however many times they tell you: how none of it is there when you're not doped up on Gnosiphen. Nothing, not even what you could have learned without SDEC,"—he pronounced it *es-dec*, the way medical students do, rather than articulating the letters—"and how worthless that makes you feel. How worthless it makes you."

"Worthless? The neurosurgery you perform in State, no one could ever be that good otherwise."

His eyes met mine. "How good does one need to be?"

Good question, but not the route I wanted to go down. My goals here were practical.

"I don't know. You started medical school, what, 11 years ago?"

"Ten."

"Ten. So you were in the third year that did the all-SDEC training. Even including the previous, partially SD cohorts, it's only been 15 years, and look how much the world has changed. Would you want to be flown by a pilot who isn't in State? Or have a Natural accountant handle your tax return?"

He just shrugged again. A small provocation should do it. "Or be operated on by a surgeon off his Gnoshiphen?"

He laughed bitterly. "We're heading there anyway. Don't you read the papers? The world's reserves of falcondoite are dwindling, and you can't make Gnosiphen without it. I don't know much, but I do understand what it means when they say there's only 10 years' worth left."

"The best chemists in the world are working on synthetic solutions."

"Oh yeah, and they're all SD too. Once the shortage hits, the whole world will be thrown into the Stone Age because no one will know how to do anything when they're not on drugs."

Strange. He didn't seem like the social crusader type. "Is that why you did it? To send the world a warning?"

A short pause. "No."

I waited. People find silence awkward. Unprepared, they tend to fill it with the truth. Eventually, he said quietly, "I just wanted to see if I could do my job as . . . me. Just me, for a change."

"And?"

"And now I know. With no enhancement, maybe I could have learned to be a neurosurgeon. But I'm not."

Fine. On to the event itself, "How long did it take you to realize that, once you started the operation?"

"No time. It was bloody obvious the moment I made the first cut."

"Why didn't you stop?"

"I couldn't. I kept hoping . . . I don't know . . . that my hands would remember what to do if I just stuck with it. Anyway, it only took a couple more minutes for the resident to put an end to the charade." He seemed fully aware of his actions and their consequences, but I needed to tick the box.

"And your surgical activity up to that point . . . "

"I'd caused a severe hematoma, obstructing access to the patient's subarachnoid tumor. Her chances of survival are severely reduced, but I'm not in State, so I can't tell you by how much."

No point asking how that made him feel. I knew the answer—could see it in his body language, hear it in his voice, even smell the specific telltale molecules in his sweat. He was not deluded, nor in denial. Bottom line, though, this wasn't really about him. Time to get at the wider implications.

"Say you hadn't had SD training. If you tried to do surgery tired or hung-over, you might screw up then too, right?" He nodded and then shrugged. I went on, "The professional thing to do is to make sure you're at your best. But how is that different from using SD enhancement to be certain that you are?"

"I don't know. It's not the same."

"How so?"

"If I could work out of State, it . . . would be me. Actually me."

Now to see how deep his insight went. "And why does that matter? In State or out of it, you're a doctor. You took an oath." He nodded, thinking, then shook his head.

Eventually, he said, "I know, but I just had to. It became an obsession."

Disappointing, but no more shallow than could be expected. I could see so much more in his posture, the timbre of his voice, the microexpressions formed by his forehead muscles. How a high need for achievement—a key criterion for selection into SD training programs—turned out to inevitably clash with the depersonalized nature of the achievements they guaranteed;

how a sense of self-efficacy no longer complemented conscientiousness but ended up redundant; and how SD security would definitely be needed, because I was suddenly aware that I already knew this, had known it for a while. I saw the evening lying ahead of me after the interview, the blue-green swirls in my own ID chip slowly turning gray as my brilliant capacity for forensic psychological analysis drained out of me; a long, dark, empty night commencing as the Gnosiphen in my bloodstream was metabolized and the State wore off.

Build Me a Memory

Nathaniel C. Cady*

Scientists and engineers have long looked to nature for inspiration. Mimicking natural phenomena such as swimming fish or flying birds has yielded some of the most revolutionary technologies on the planet. One of the most complex natural systems, the brain, rivals the most advanced computing technologies available today. The brain accomplishes this feat by massive parallel processing of information and extremely efficient energy use during operation. To significantly advance existing computational technology, engineers are now looking to the brain for inspiration. Aided by advances in nanotechnology, a new breed of electronic devices has been developed. These devices, known as memory resistors or memristors, occupy a unique niche in the world of electronic circuits. A hybrid between a traditional resistor and a transistor, these devices can hold "memories" indefinitely and can be switched on and off at will. Similar to neural synapses in our brains, memristors respond to electrical stimulus but only form a memory when a certain threshold is crossed. Because memristors can be built at the nanometer (one-billionth of a meter)-size scale, one can imagine vast arrays that could store memories or process information similar to that of the human brain. This technology is poised to enable "neuromorphic" computing, which closely mimics the processes of our brains. Coupled with recent advances in brain–computer interfaces, we are now facing a bold new world of computers that think like us and could even become part of us.

JOHN LOOKED AT HIS watch. How could it be just 30 seconds from the last time he had looked? It seemed like an eternity

*College of Nanoscale Science and Engineering, SUNY Polytechnic Institute, Albany, NY 12203, USA. ncady@uamail.albany.edu

unwound every minute he waited. As he drifted back to another monumental pause, a thought flickered. Wasn't this the same place he had waited last year? Wasn't it just about the same time? Why couldn't he put his finger on it?

As he dutifully observed the monotony of the white-painted space in front of him, John continued to dwell on the similarities between his current situation and the one he couldn't quite remember. *Ah hell*, he thought, *I might as well access the chip*. Reaching behind his ear, John toggled the small gray switch, wincing slightly as the electrodes fired. Nothing happened for a few seconds, but then the aura began. In a hazy mixture of soft light and amorphous sound, images started to shutter past. Like old reels of film, they started out jumpy but soon settled into a regular rhythm, grinding out his memories from the past year. He wished he had paid the premium cost for the chip with search functionality. Unfortunately, his was a second-generation chip, and scrolling through the entire set of memories was the only option. It pleased him, though, to churn through the past year. Jumping from day to day, month to month, he lost himself in the condensed, fast-forward of these visual recordings. *Damn, if there couldn't be sound to go with it.*

In the room behind the white wall, the small boy clicked together Legos at an alarming pace. One hand reached to the bucket of pieces, while the other quickly contorted the growing structure for proper placement of the next piece. Each step, each piece was perfectly in order, perfectly positioned. In minutes, the assembled structure stood before the boy, seemingly waiting for play. The boy evaluated the structure, blinked as if to clear his thoughts, and then dipped his hand into the bucket for a new round of pieces.

John got to his summer memories and forced the movie reel to reduce its pace. He remembered this section clearly, their trip to Lake Champlain. As the series of images panned around their campsite, he remembered the smell of the campfire, the repetitive sounds of waves on the shore, and the warmth of the late afternoon sun. What he hadn't remembered, at least not in his regular memory, was the way the boy had looked at him that day. Unlike so many days before, the boy came to him with a look of sheer happiness. It was a carefree look, the look of a boy unleashed on the outdoors, pocketknife in hand, ready for adventure. As the images of the boy continued, John conjured his own boyhood memories of camping. How similar he and the boy had been, at least in this moment.

The boy reached into the bucket and realized that he had taken the last piece. He was five pieces away from finishing the new structure. Where were the missing pieces? The image clearly showed steps 37 to 41, and those steps required one piece per step. Where were they? He blinked repeatedly. His brow dampened. The twitch started. A few squints in the left eye, head cocking to the side, the boy looked as if he was straining to focus his eyesight. Looking around the room he could see 12 other structures, all slightly different, arranged almost as a small town. Where were those missing pieces? Maybe he had added too many to one of the other structures. But how could he have added too many? The instructions clearly showed every step, every piece. His shirt was now damp. The twitch was nearly continuous now. Where were those pieces?

John was at the end of the camping trip. The last few images showed the boy packing bags into the car and hopping into the passenger seat. The car door closed, and John knew he needed to get back to his task. Scrolling faster, he got into the fall and the start of school for the boy. *Ah, getting warmer.* This had to be the right time frame. Wasn't this about the time they made the last trip to . . .

"Mr. Fitch?"

"Yes, that's me."

"Please step into my office, we have made some developments on your son's implant."

John's quick transition from the memory movie to verbal communication gave him an instant headache. Why were these chips so unobtrusive when they collected memories but so annoying when retrieving? He again wished he had opted for the premium model. Oh well, might as well find out what the doctor had come up with. Stepping into the doctor's office, John noted the lack of paper, decorations, or just about anything of note, except for the large computer monitor on the desk. Leaning forward, the doctor gave John a curious look.

"John, your son's implant has integrated better than nearly any implant we have placed in a child of his age. His cognitive reasoning is off the charts, and his combined natural and augmented memory is well above average. To put it bluntly, he is functioning like a child at least five years older." John shrugged, "So what's the problem then?"

"Well, it is actually difficult to measure. You see, we have plenty of ways to measure cognitive ability and memory retention, but we have no way of quantifying play?"

"Huh," snorted John. "What do you mean, quantifying play?"

"Well, I don't really know how to put it."

"Put what?"

"Your son doesn't seem to enjoy playing."

"How can you tell?"

"That's the thing, it's not something I can quantify. It's just a feeling that I have, actually all of us here at the center have, after observing your son."

"That's ridiculous."

"I understand how it must sound, but have you watched the boy?"

"Of course I watch him. I'm with him every day. He plays for hours."

"Does he smile when he plays?"

"He's usually building with Legos. He is always very concentrated."

"Is he proud of the structures he builds?"

"Well . . ." John thought about this last question. Did the boy ever show him the finished structures? Was he excited about them? Was he ever excited about anything?

"John, we think your son may be utilizing his memristive memory and neuromorphic cognition to such an extent that he is neglecting some of the natural portions of his brain."

"You must be kidding. The memristive implant is supposed to enhance his thinking and memory. How could it detract from his natural mind?"

"This is certainly the first case we have seen like this, but your son is also one of the youngest patients to receive an implant and one of the most successful at integrating it with his natural brain. We're actually concerned that he has become so well integrated that he has forgotten to access some his natural thought processes and pleasure centers."

John thought about this for a moment. Could it be true? Could the boy be so well integrated that he simply forgot how to have fun? He thought about his own implant, the clunky old version with only linear memory recall and the painful startup shock. He was integrated but only in the sense that he could access memories and do quick calculations, when needed. He wasn't really integrated. What if he could call up distinct memories, instruction manuals, recipes, directions, or even names and phone numbers on a whim? Would it be different? Would he be able to let go or turn it off?

"John, we want you to try something with your son."

"What is it?"

"Can you remember a time when he looked happy, when he seemed carefree and just plain happy?"

"Yes."

"Can you describe that time?"

John thought of the camping trip. He was tempted to switch on the chip, to recreate the image of the boy's happy face. He resisted. He dug into his own memory, his natural memory, and summoned the smells, the sounds, the warmth, the boy.

"John, are you still with me?"

"Sorry, I was just recalling the time we went camping, just last year. It was summer. We were on Lake Champlain. He was so happy. I remember his face. He looked like a kid on the last day of school."

"Do you think you can recreate that trip?"

"Sure, it's still August. I'm sure we could get a campsite."

"We think that you need to bring him back into that moment, to give him that same feeling of happiness, so he can access that portion of his brain. We don't think you should shut down his implant's functioning but, instead, augment the memristive memories and cognition with his own natural memories, pleasures, and thought processes."

"That makes him sound like more of a robot than a boy."

"John, in some ways, the memristor chip has given him the ability to be a hybrid. His brain has learned to use both its own functions and the memristive chip functions, but since he's a child, he isn't able to balance these functions in the same way as you and me."

As John mulled this over, he thought of his first cell phone and his first smart phone. What had he done before he had instant access to phone chats and the Internet? Wasn't it funny that he could no longer remember his schedule for the next day, much less a month from now? How dependent had he become on this external device, which he could simply leave in his pocket? He was an adult by the time he got his first smart phone, and so even as connected as he had become, he still could shut it off. What if he had always had it?

"John, I feel like I've lost you again."

"Oh, sorry, I was just thinking about my first smart phone."

"Are you thinking of how dependent you became?"

"Yes, and those weren't even implanted."

"No, they weren't. But look how dependent we all became on them. Just imagine having our memristive implants from childhood. How much more would we depend on them?" John blinked a few times and then slowly extended his hand. "Thank you, doctor. I think you may be right."

As they shook hands, John began thinking of the campsite. Walking down the hallway to the boy's room, he once again noted the expanse of white-painted wall. He stopped abruptly. That was it, the white walls, the long hallway, all of the white trim. He hadn't gotten this far in his memory movie, but it was there, right at the cusp of his natural memory. And then he had it. It was the waiting room outside the school office in the second month of school. It was so clear now. He remembered the principal and the guidance counselor talking about the tests. The boy had scored so well they wanted to move him into the next grade. He remembered being so proud of the boy, so pleased with the performance of the implant. But he also remembered worrying that skipping grades would make things awkward for the boy. He worried about his friends. Who would he play with in the next grade? Would the kids be nice to him?

Chapter 10

Who Do They Think They Are?

Reginald H. Garrett
Department of Biology, Physical Life Sciences Building (PLSB),
University of Virginia, 90 Geldard Drive, Charlottesville, VA 22903, USA
rhg@virginia.edu

What is race? The United States Census Bureau census form asks people to self-identify, offering a choice of 15 boxes to check, beginning with *White, Black, American Indian*, followed by an additional 11 (one of which is *Filipino*; another is *Guamanian or Chamorro*), and concluding with one labeled *Some Other Race*. None of the 15 offers a choice of *Hispanic, Latino*, or any other accepted term used by US residents whose ethnic heritage links them to countries in Central or South America. Odd, given the preoccupation both political parties show toward this ethnic group. Although the lack of a Latino box is puzzling, it is apparent that the Census Bureau is treading lightly here, hoping to avoid offending anyone. And, Hispanics tend to self-identify as white. As we know all too well, race can be a very contentious matter. The general, and reasonable, assumption is that genetic differences underlie race.

Creating Life from Life: Biotechnology and Science Fiction
Edited by Rosalyn W. Berne
Copyright © 2015 Pan Stanford Publishing Pte. Ltd.
ISBN 978-981-4463-58-4 (Hardcover), 978-981-4463-59-1 (eBook)
www.panstanford.com

Biological science defines race as "a group with internal similarity that distinguishes it from other groups." The genetic definition of each of us is our uniquely personal DNA. Much of the differences between us can be ascribed to differences in our DNA, but these differences are, quantitatively speaking, trivial. After all, the genetic differences between chimpanzees and humans, whose lineages diverged six or seven million years ago, is less than 1.4%. So we should not expect human groups to show very much genetic variation. As a matter of fact, the greatest genetic difference between any two randomly chosen humans is 0.1% or less. Of this 0.1%, only 6% or so (i.e., 0.006%) accounts for those observable features that we use to pigeonhole people by race, things like skin color or facial characteristics—such as the breadth of a person's nose. In actuality, there are no sharp racial distinctions; humans form a continuum of overt appearances and underlying genetic differences. The human species is, despite the consternation caused, promiscuous. "Genetic purity" is a myth.

The people populating the world today are descendants of a group of *Homo sapiens* termed "modern humans" by anthropologists. These modern humans originated in sub-Saharan Africa. Groups of them left Africa around 60,000 years ago, and their subsequent migrations over the ensuing 40,000–50,000 years have populated the far corners of the globe (Wade, 2006). Some even mated with Neanderthals, an earlier strain of humans living in Eurasia. Children were born of these sexual unions, verified by the vestiges of Neanderthal DNA found in all extant humans descended from ancestors living outside Africa. Humans alive today whose ancestors stayed in Africa bear no such traces of Neanderthal DNA (Green et al., 2010). So much for the egregiously stupid claims of "racial purity" touted by anyone.

The most obvious trait used to classify human race is skin color. Western civilization has been haunted by its predilection to organize itself around this meaningless marker. Martin Luther King, Jr., so pointedly and poignantly exposed the fallacy of this prejudice when he dreamt that his children might ". . . one day live in a nation where they will not be judged by the color of their skin but by the content of their character" (King, 1963) Yet the mindless notion that desirable human qualities—intelligence, integrity, honor, courage, and too many more—are roughly apportioned along some scale where white is superior and black is inferior remains perniciously difficult to dislodge. What is the biological basis of the Caucasian coloring, a common attribute among those prone to arrogate to themselves all desirable attributes?

Even the earliest Africans had black skin. It provides essential protection from the cancerous ultraviolet (UV) radiation of the tropical sun. The pigment responsible is melanin. As a heritable trait, melanin production is encoded in our DNA. Humans who migrated to northern Europe gradually experienced a decline in melanin levels as an adaptation to their environment. At higher latitudes, sunlight is weak, and the risk of skin cancer is less. Melanin production no longer poses much advantage; instead, it actually becomes a disadvantage because melanin diminishes vitamin D production in the skin. The phrase "sunshine vitamin D" reminds of this benefit of sunlight, because UV-B irradiation drives the conversion of 7-dehydrocholesterol located in the deep layers of the skin into pre-vitamin D3, which spontaneously changes into vitamin D. Melanin absorbs UV-B, preventing it from reaching 7-dehydrocholesterol. Black skin contains three to six times as much melanin as fair skin. About 25% of the UV-B light passes through the epidermis of fair skin, but only 7% or so UV-B gets through black skin (Brenner and Hearing, 2008). Vitamin D deficiency leads to rickets, a nutritional disease characterized by softening of the bones and crippling deformities. Such skeletal weaknesses would lead to a decline in fitness of individuals producing melanin, and natural selection would favor fair-skinned individuals whose vitamin D production was not impaired. That is, chance mutations that limited melanin biosynthesis gave individuals living at high latitudes a selective advantage. So, lighter skin color evolved and became fixed in northern European populations because it provided for better vitamin D synthesis and the avoidance of rickets, a debilitating disease.

Recent research in human genetics has identified four genes underlying human skin pigmentation (Norton et al., 2007). One of these genes accounts for about one-third of skin color differences (Lamason et al., 2005); it encodes a protein necessary for melanosome formation. Melanosomes are the subcellular structures that house melanin. The gene has two variant forms. Nearly all Africans and East Asians carry the ancestral variant of the gene. On the other hand, 98% of Europeans carry the mutant form. The emergence of this genetic change among European populations has been dated to between 11,000 and 19,000 years ago (Beleza et al., 2012). The difference in the protein produced by the two gene forms seems trivial. Only one amino acid change occurs in the precise order of the 500 amino acids that define this protein. In the ancestral gene, the amino acid alanine occurs at position 111 in the amino acid sequence. Alanine is defined by its $-CH_3$ side chain. In the mutant form of the gene, threonine replaces alanine. Threonine's side chain is $-C(HOH)-CH_3$. Pause to consider: The prejudice that spawned innumerable human tragedies can in large measure be traced back to this seemingly minor difference of a few atoms among the 10,000 or so that constitute this one protein.

Might this melanosome-forming gene help us in classifying humans by race? Not really. Were we to classify humans according to race in any scientifically valid way, we would have to consider the variation in more than just this one gene; indeed, we would have to look at hundreds of genes, perhaps more. How many human genes are there, and can we look at all of them across a representative sample of the entire human population? The Human Genome Project, a multinational research endeavor to decipher the totality of the genetic information in a human individual, began in 1990 and was completed in 2003, at a total cost of $3 billion, or about $1 for each of the three billion base pairs of DNA that constitute the human genome. (How big is three billion base pairs—the pairs of structural units in the DNA double helix? These base pairs can be equated with letters. The Bible contains somewhat over 3.5 million letters, so the human genome is nine times larger than the Bible.) This research accomplishment gave a surprising result—the human genome contains just slightly more than 20,000 genes, or only a fifth as many as experts expected. Our marvelously textured and exquisitely layered complexity derives from how these 20,000 genes are expressed, not so much from how many there are.

It may surprise the reader to discover that, despite this great number of base pairs and these many genes, biotechnology has given us tools that can make quantitative comparisons between the genomes of any 2 individuals or, indeed, between nearly 1000 individuals from all over the map; it has been done (Li et al., 2008). Using such global genomic tools, we focus out from the fine structure of a single amino acid change in one gene and instead compare more than 650,000 genetic indicators across a representative sample of humanity—981 individuals from 51 populations scattered around the world (Li et al., 2008). Such studies were spawned to probe the genetic basis of human disease, but they also illuminate relationships between the origins and geographical distribution of human populations. The results confirm that humans evolved in sub-Saharan Africa and migrated to every corner of the world, adapting to a wide diversity of habitats and climates. The results also reveal that reproductive isolation of human populations took place through the geographical boundaries that separated them from one another. Simply put, until recently, people didn't travel much, and they procreated with neighbors, giving rise to genetically distinct subpopulations defined by geography. These different populations have distinct genetic profiles that correlate with six major geographical regions: Africa, Europe and the Middle East, South Asia, Oceania, East Asia, and the Americas (specifically, Amerindians). Historically, geography has been and remains an important determinant of human evolutionary history (Wang, Zöllner, and Rosenberg, 2012). The mobility of humans in the 21st century will likely blur these boundaries over time.

So, when we compare the genomes of randomly chosen individuals, the genetic differences seem trivial. When we stand back and probe deeply for genetic differences between geographically defined populations, we can find differences that correlate with geography. It makes sense. Genetic diversity within a species has a fascinating attribute: Genetic diversity is greater in the location where the species first evolved, that is, where the founding population of the species arose. This principle explains why the genetic diversity within a single sub-Saharan tribe is greater than the genetic diversity found among the many representatives from nearly 200 member countries around the world who work in the United Nations building in New York. From the correlation of geography with genetic difference, it follows obviously that the visible evidence of human genetic variation provides those bent on racial discrimination with sufficient features on which to hang their appearance-based bias. The fallacy lies in conflating these differences with hierarchal notions of value. There is no scientific evidence to support insidious generalities of this nature.

The proposition that geographically isolated human populations (Africans, Asians, Europeans) may have experienced divergent evolution in social behavior seems valid (Wade, 2014). That the social behavior of different populations followed different evolutionary paths is to be expected as these people were shaped by the challenges of their particular environment. Further, these behavioral variations may explain the emergence of different social institutions that favored greater (or less) economic or military success (Wade, 2014). Even so, what remains truly striking about human genetics is that we are more or less the same. This being so, we might find greater truth and satisfaction in celebrating our sameness, rather than extolling the things that distinguish us and our kin from others. The spectrum of human differences is splendid and fertile, but these distinctions are mostly cultural, not so much biological.

Celebrating diversity emphasizes (or should) these ethnic and cultural distinctions, not racial ones. Biology informs us that celebrations of diversity are worthy when they tell us who we are, as long as we use such differences to focus on us, but such celebrations lose their value, indeed become unacceptable, when they become an excuse to criticize, to marginalize, or, worse, to persecute others.

References

Beleza, S., Santos, A. M., McEvoy, B., Alves, I., Martinho, C., Cameron, E., . . . and Rocha, J. (2012). The timing of pigmentation lightening in Europeans. *Molecular Biology and Evolution*. doi:10.1093/molbev/mss207.

Brenner, M., and Hearing, V. J. (2008). The protective role of melanin against UV damage in human skin. *Photochemistry and Photobiology*, **84**, 539–549.

Green, R. E., Krause, J., Briggs. A. W, Tomislav, M., Udo, S., Kircher, M., . . . and Pääbo, S. (2010). A draft sequence of the Neanderthal genome. *Science*, **328**, 710–722.

King, M. L., Jr. (1963, August 28). *I Have a Dream*. Speech from the steps of the Lincoln Memorial, Washington, DC.

Lamason, R. L., Mohideen, M.-A. P. K., Mest, J. R., Wong, A. C., Norton, H. L., Aros, M. C., . . . and Cheng, K. C. (2005). SLC24A5, a putative cation exchanger, affects pigmentation in zebrafish and humans. *Science*, **310**, 1782–1786.

Li, J. Z., Absher, D. M., Tang, H., Southwick, A. M., Casto, A. M., Ramachandran, S., . . . and Myers, R. M. (2008). Worldwide human relationships inferred from genome-wide patterns of variation. *Science*, **319**, 1100–1104.

Norton, H. L., Kittles, R. A., Parra, E., McKeigue, P., Mao, X., Cheng, K., . . . and Shriver, M. D. (2007). Genetic evidence for the convergent evolution of light skin in Europeans and East Asians. *Molecular Biology and Evolution*, **24**, 710–722.

Wade, N. (2006). *Before the Dawn: Recovering the Lost History of Our Ancestors.* New York, NY: The Penguin Press.

Wade, N. (2014). *A Troublesome Inheritance: Genes, Race and Human History.* New York, NY: The Penguin Press.

Wang, C., Zöllner, S., and Rosenberg, N. A. (2012). A quantitative comparison of the similarity between genes and geography in worldwide human populations. *PLoS Genetics*, **8**, e1002886. doi:10.1371/journal.pgen.1002886.

Emmanuel

Rosalyn W. Berne

This is an edited excerpt from the science fiction novel Waiting in the Silence. *The setting is a near-term future on the island of Nantucket, where the Virtual Information System for Human Noetic Evolution and Welfare (VISHNEW) has emerged. Exquisitely intelligent, it appears to have formed independent of human design. Emmanuel, an island resident who is connected to VISHNEW, benefits from the enhancements it provides. Unfortunately, his friend Oriana does not. But as a child rejected by his own parents for his genetic anomaly, even an enhanced life of VISHNEW connection cannot overcome Emmanuel's personal torment.*

EMMANUEL AND HIS MOTHER and father have just returned home. Oriana pours a beverage into a tall glass and heads quickly out the kitchen door. "You can come over here to my house if you want," Oriana yells across the lawn to a Hood friend she has never actually met in person. "Here's some lemonade!" Emmanuel turns when he hears her voice. He looks as if he wants to reply to her invitation. "Well, are you coming over or not?" Oriana shouts. Emmanuel drops his gaze toward the ground. "Oh, come on," she chides, holding the glass out in front of her. Emmanuel steps toward her with the soft deliberation of a cautious yet curious kitten. "You're going to like it," she assures him. "This crop of lemons is especially sweet."

Emmanuel gently places one foot after another on the dew-soaked ground, causing a squishing squeaky sound with each step. Oriana holds out the tall, ice-filled cup as he approaches, and the boy accepts it with a placid grin.

Emmanuel sips the drink, crossing his eyes as he studies the floating ice. Oriana sees nothing wrong with him at all. She likes him, even though she finds him a bit aloof and disinterested.

"Come on, let's sit down," Oriana invites.

Emmanuel and Oriana take seats on the upper step of Oriana and Papa's home. Oriana looks at her friend with a wide grin, not quite sure what to make of him. The boy stares out at the clearing across the road, to what was once a grove of loblolly pines, before the moths shredded them of their life force, and the Great Storms brought their roots up out of the ground. He slurps down the remainder of his lemonade.

"What's so interesting over there?" Oriana asks him. Emmanuel shrugs. She watches him closely as he stares at nothing that Oriana can fathom.

For nearly an hour they sit saying nothing at all. At times Emmanuel taps his knee. At other times he puts his hand on her shoulder or her thigh for a few moments. Then, for no apparent reason, Emmanuel gets up and heads back home.

The boy looks over his shoulder, making brief eye contact with the only friend he has. . . .

. . . A few weeks later, Oriana spots Emmanuel coming toward the front door of her home.

"Hey!" Oriana yells to him. "Do you want to go for a walk with me?"

"OK," Emmanuel says mumbling, suddenly appearing right in front of her.

She can hardly believe he's offering to spend time with her. But there aren't many walking other than into the center of town and back, strolling down Main Street to the old wharf, heading out past the Whaling Museum near Granddad's house, or climbing along the dike.

"To the tree," he says, drumming his fingers on her shoulder.

"Tree? What tree?" Oriana inquires. She assumes he is suggesting a game involving an imaginary tree.

"Oh," she says pointing across the street. She giggles, still unsure of herself in his physical presence. She hasn't yet learned how to interpret all the nuances of his expressions. "You must be talking about that huge white pine over there, the one with the low branches we can climb," she says pointing to a nearby meadow. Emmanuel removes his hand from her shoulder.

"No," he mumbles, dropping his eyes to the ground. Oriana sighs, placing her hand on his hand. She didn't mean to mock or disappoint him.

"Come on, Emmanuel, what tree are you talking about then?" she asks.

"From my dream," he replies in a whisper.

"Dream?" she asks. Oriana is puzzled.

Emmanuel heads across the street, in the opposite direction from him home. Then he takes off running across the empty lot.

"Hey!" Oriana yells following, moving her adolescent legs at as fast a run as she can. "Slow down, will you!" she yells as he crosses the clearing and turns left onto the next street. When he finally stops, the two are standing in front of a bright-blue hover-scooter parked on the side of the road. "Whose is this?" she asks, panting, as she catches up to Emmanuel.

"Don't know," he answers, climbing onto the vehicle.

Oriana, still engrossed in what she surmises to be an imagination game, gets on behind Emmanuel and wraps her arms around his waist.

"Let's go to a magical forest where the trees are huge and full of life," she suggests, closing her eyes to create the vision in her mind.

Emmanuel starts the engine.

"Hey, what are you doing?" Oriana exclaims. "I'm not allowed to ride on these. Anyway, we'll get into huge trouble."

Emmanuel shifts into launch mode on a machine designed for both air and ground transportation. Shaped like an oblong dish with wheels, the vehicle has a windshield and a seat built for two, and its stealth motion makes barely a whisper as it glides upward through the air. The control mechanism is a touch-sensitive panel on the windshield, displaying "Forward," "Lift," "Lower," "Slow," and "Stop." It is simple to operate. The machine rather than its driver regulates the speed, as prompted by variable conditions such as traffic flow, wind, and the sunlight that provides it power. Emmanuel and Oriana head out from Orange Street onto Polpis Road, gliding over what the Great Storms have left of Quaise Pastures.

"This isn't a walk," Oriana exclaims over the cat-like purr of the engine.

"Yahoo!" Emmanuel shouts with glee as they soar further away from town and out over the desolate terrain. When they land, it is between two swaths of thick, brown scrub.

"A bog?" Oriana asks in amazement.

Emmanuel hops off the craft and takes off running for the edge of the thicket.

Oriana wishes he would take her by the hand or say something or at least look back to know that she was still there. "Slow down, Emmanuel," she shouts breathlessly, jogging tentatively behind the boy. Emmanuel raises his arms over his head, as if mimicking flight.

Back in the early part of the twenty-first century, the Masquetuck Reservation was a 14-acre nature preserve of both native and non-native flora. Three-quarters of a century later, it is overrun with scrub oaks and an entanglement of vines growing up and over the remaining stubs of once robust deciduous trees and conifers. Kudzu, wisteria, a hearty variety of stinging nettle, and other aggressive non-native species had worked their way through the stumps and rot of what used to be a mature forest grove.

Emmanuel yanks at the encroaching vines, unveiling a rugged path through the overgrowth of late spring. Slowing his gait to accommodate the changing terrain, he pushes through briars, thistle, and robust shoots of poison oak as he moves to the commands of an untamed will. Oriana trails hopelessly behind.

When finally Oriana catches up, she finds her friend standing under a magnificent white oak. Huge by comparison to any tree Oriana has ever seen.

"Wow, this one must be pretty old," she remarks. "I wonder how big it is." Trying to estimate its height Oriana gazes up to its top, framing her fingers into a square and peering through them as she extends her arm outward. The change in perception fails to provide the information she needs to make more than a random guess at its size.

"Well, if size is what you're trying to figure out, I can give you an exact measurement of both its width and its height," Emmanuel blurts out, using more words than she's heard him speak all day. "I can gauge it to within a centimeter of accuracy and even convert it into the English customary system," he continues.

The opal yellow of a VISHNEW-enhanced focus washes over Emmanuel's eyes. He moves his gaze from treetop to roots. "It's 48.75 feet tall," he answers.

"Damn, you sure do think you're smart," Oriana mumbles under her breath. He may be trying to impress her, but it's humiliating. "Well, what's its circumference, Emmanuel?" she asks, hoping he won't be able to come up with the answer and wishing the humiliation would end. Oriana feels stupid for the first time in her life.

"How do you think this tree survived the Great Storms?" she inquires, hoping to impress him with her knowledge of historical events. Emmanuel doesn't acknowledge the question. Instead, he plops down on the ground and pulls off his shoes. Rubbing his bare soles on the loamy soil, he twists and turns them in the dirt with a purpose. Oriana sits down next to him and pounds her shoe-covered feet against the trunk of the tree.

"Stop that," Emmanuel scolds her. "How would you like to be treated that way?"

Oriana notices his dirty feet, clumps of soil between his toes. "Yuck," she exclaims, pointing at them. Emmanuel lifts a foot and rubs it against her bare leg.

"Hey, stop it!" she fusses as he laughs. He shoves his other foot against her calf.

The boy stands, and steps over an exposed root. Leaning his body against the trunk of the tree he wraps his arms around it as much as he is able and slides his body up and down along the bark. Oriana steps back in disgust. She may still be young, but Oriana knows enough about boys to suspect she is witnessing some kind of sexual perversion. And to make matters worse, Emmanuel begins to hum and moan, sliding his hands along the jagged bark and pressing his face against its surface.

"Why are you doing that?" she asks.

"You should come try so you can feel it, too," Emmanuel invites her.

Oriana shakes her head, the soft ripples of her shoulder-length brown hair moving sideways with the motion. She is anxious and fears that actually touching the tree could cause her harm.

"Oh, come on," he teases. His plea she disregards. It is her own curiosity that finally compels her.

"Feel what?" she asks, tentatively stepping closer to the trunk.

"I can't tell you what it is. You have to feel it is all. Like me; do like I'm doing."

"Fine then," she replies, stretching her arms around the trunk. Before her face touches the bark, she scans the tree's surface for mites, lichen, or small vines that could lead to contact dermatitis. Oriana leans in further to make full-body contact with the tree's thick mass. No harm seems to be come to her as a result.

"Do you feel it?" Emmanuel asks, the pitch of his voice rising a bit. She has no idea what he is talking about.

"It's rigid and hard. Sort of rough," she huffs.

"No, I mean do you feel the tree?"

"I don't get what you're asking," she offers, longing to know what sort of sensations he might be experiencing.

"Well, maybe for you it would be better to turn around and try to feel it through your back." Oriana follows his suggestion, pressing her spine along a vertical protrusion in the trunk. "Why are you holding your head forward like that?" he asks her, tapping his foot in annoyance. "Go ahead and put your head against the tree. Make your whole body touch, or you won't feel it," Emmanuel instructs.

She leans closer to the tree, resting her head against the bark. When she imagines something crawling in her hair Oriana begins to squirm. "Calm down or it won't work," Emmanuel instructs. Oriana convinces herself that the crawling sensation is only her imagination and continues to hold on to the tree.

"Now let go," he instructs her.

"Let go?" she asks, as she begins to finally to relax. "If I let go, I might fall."

"No, not of the tree, of yourself. Let go of yourself, and then maybe you'll be able to feel it all the way." Once again she tries to imagine what Emmanuel feels. Pushing past the tears of frustration that are welling up inside of her eyes, she attempts to let herself go.

"I'm alive," Emmanuel cries out suddenly, his voice carried upward along the branches in vocal vibrations aiming for the sky.

"Of course you are," she hollers in return.

"I am alive!" he cries out, louder than before.

"Me too!" she sings out.

Oriana hops up onto a low branch and hangs upside-down from the great tree. The blood rushes into her brain as she hangs. She begins to sense something unusual in herself. Releasing the tree trunk, Emmanuel lies down on the ground, wraps his arms around his knees, and curls into a ball. Oriana turns her attention to her friend, who lies motionless on the ground, her perception askew being upside-down.

"What are you doing down there?" she asks slipping off the branch to find herself curled up next to Emmanuel.

"What time is it?" she inquires, concerned that Papa must be really upset by now. She doubts her remote connection is working at all this far out and surmises that Papa is bound to be growing anxious, since he has no idea of her whereabouts.

Emmanuel sits up and lifts a hand to his forehead. "Hmm," he sounds. "Do you want Eastern Standard time, with the daylight saving factor from the Nantucket Town clock? Or would you prefer the Coordinated Universal Time from the Cesium Fountain Atomic Clock in Boulder, Colorado?" Oriana yanks hard on his left earlobe.

"Could you stop being such a jerk and just tell me whatever time Papa has now?"

"Ouch," he complains.

"Well? What time is it?" she asks again.

"It sounds like you want to know if it's time for us to go home. To which the answer is probably 'yes.' It's been 138 minutes since we left your steps."

"We'd better go," she suggests.

The two make their way back through the thicket, wordless, hand in hand. The ride home on the hover-scooter is peaceful, a barely perceptible breeze rocking the craft slightly from front to back as they glide. The vehicle lands itself exactly in the place where they found it.

A few weeks later Emmanuel and his mother stand on Oriana's front steps. The two are locked arm in arm. A man who Oriana assumes to be the boy's father stands closely behind the pair.

"Oriana, does your father know about your little adventure with Emmanuel?" the woman asks, raising her left eyebrow. She interrupts Oriana's attempt at a reply. "We do not approve of this friendship," the woman declares, lifting her index finger toward Oriana and scowling.

"We need to speak with Gardiner," the man tells Oriana as he pushes his way toward the open door. The man has blond hair like Emmanuel's, only much thinner and with flakes of dead skin caught in some of the front strands. He reaches for bangs that partially obscure his eyes, pulling his hair across his forehead and behind his ears to reveal the telling tiny scar at each of his temples. *Connected, of course*, Oriana acknowledges.

"Sure, I'll go in and get him," she replies, stepping inside her home. Papa appears at that moment and greets the unexpected guests, welcoming them inside.

"What a surprise," Papa remarks to his neighbors as they enter the foyer.

"My mate and I are here to ensure that the boy and Oriana will not be socializing anymore," the woman explains.

"But why not?" Oriana protests from inside the foyer. "That's not fair!"

Papa gestures for them to take a seat on the living room couch. Emmanuel's mother seats Emmanuel between his father and herself. Papa's face folds into scorn.

"We have no choice, really," the boy's father exclaims.

Emmanuel gazes through the panes of the triple-hung windows.

"Then how will we stay best friends?" Oriana implores, tears streaming from her eyes. "We only just met in person for the first time!"

Emmanuel props his feet onto the couch, clutching his knees in his arms. A clump of hair falls across his eyes. Papa takes notice of the boy's appearance: smooth, dark skin, the blue side of black; light yellow hair bordering on platinum; and pale, very pale blue eyes. He considers what an interesting set of design selections these parents have made for their only child.

"How about if I stay with them whenever Emmanuel comes to visit?" Papa suggests.

Oriana's face lights up, her eyes twinkling with adoration. He knows this is her only friend and how much she cares about him.

"I don't think so," Emmanuel's father says as he stands. "We should go," he says to his mate.

In a little less than an hour, Emmanuel's mother returns. Papa spots her face pressed against the colorful windowpanes as he passes from the kitchen to the stairs.

"Come in, please," he offers, opening the door. "May I offer you a cup of tea?" Papa smiles, gesturing her toward the kitchen, where she sits down at the table, her back rigid against the chair, her feet perched on its lowest rung. Oriana sits down beside her.

Emmanuel's mother sips the warm, sweet drink with two hands. "Mmm," she says. "You make a nice cup of tea." Chin on hand, elbow propped firmly on the table, Oriana stares at her friend's mother. Papa also focuses on the woman before him, who he finds unattractively pale, too frail, and annoyingly timid.

"What exactly are you doing here? What is it that you want?" Papa asks of Emmanuel's mother.

"I feel like I can confide in you," she replies, her head dropping a bit, her eyes focused on the cup of tea in her hands.

"What do you mean?" Papa asks. "Confide in me about what?"

"We had no idea he'd come out like this."

"Who? Like what?"

"All we wanted was to protect the child from ultraviolet exposure," she explains. "It's so dangerous for pale-complexioned children these days. We only wanted to keep him safe. It's that, well . . ."

"Well, what?"

"Oh," she replies, lost in thought. "It frightened me terribly."

"What frightened you?"

"The boy, of course," she elaborates. "How can you not have noticed?'

Papa shrugs. "You mean his skin color?"

The woman nods. "When they put it in my arms I didn't know what to do. No one warned us. As you can imagine, I thought, 'How could this be mine? How could this have come from inside of my womb?' At first I didn't want it."

"If you are talking about Emmanuel, I think you mean to say 'him'. You didn't want *him*."

"I was never so startled in my life." Emmanuel's mother turns her focus to a dying spider plant hanging in the kitchen window. "We thought it best to keep him in our home," she continues, "out of the direct view of other islanders. Somehow, 16 years went by before we finally let him out."

"Are you saying that Emmanuel had been inside his house his entire life? Papa asks in amazement. The woman keeps talking, paying no attention to Papa's interjections of "What? What did you say?"

"I didn't mean to hurt him. Really, I didn't. I was trying to explain things to him the best I could."

"I can appreciate that," Papa reassures her.

"Recently we let him out like he wanted. Now something has gone terribly wrong," she announces.

"Apparently," Papa says. "What is his prognosis?"

"Not so good if he continues to venture outside into the public domain," she responds.

"They have a special friendship, you know," Papa offers.

Emmanuel's mother clears her throat and places the nail of an index finger between her teeth. She gnaws the nail until the skin beneath it bleeds. A wordless moment passes between them.

"You ought to consider his emotional needs," Papa scolds.

Abruptly Emmanuel's mother heads out the kitchen door. Oriana watches as the woman marches down the steps, across the side yard, into the front door of her own house. Within a few minutes the mother returns to the side door with Emmanuel by her side.

"So you're back!" he says to the pair.

The panther-complexioned teenager with blond hair and clear blue eyes pulls his hand out of his mother's clutch and sits at the table beside his friend.

"Only one more chance. That's it," his mother scolds. "If anything at all goes wrong, that's it for Emmanuel and Oriana's so-called friendship. Back into the house he will go."

"One more chance," Oriana mumbles as her friend's mother gets up to leave. The woman shuts the door with a bang.

Chapter 11

The Uncertain Consequences of the Biotechnology Revolution

Catherine Rhodes

Institute for Science, Ethics and Innovation, Faculty of Life Sciences,
University of Manchester, Oxford Road, Manchester,
M13 9PL, UK
catherine.rhodes-2@manchester.ac.uk

The biotechnology revolution has involved a major technological change—a move to the new ability to understand and manipulate life forms at the genetic level. All major technological changes have social and economic consequences, and because of the breadth of applications of modern biotechnology, the socioeconomic consequences will be many and diverse. It promises a new level of control over our environment and us. There are many positive consequences to this. Human health can be improved through better understanding, treatment, and prevention of disease. New solutions can be found to some of our environmental problems with alternative sources of energy, cleaner manufacturing processes, and new means of reducing pollution. Novel agricultural technologies can provide crops with enhanced or novel traits, reducing inputs, improving nutritional

Creating Life from Life: Biotechnology and Science Fiction
Edited by Rosalyn W. Berne
Copyright © 2015 Pan Stanford Publishing Pte. Ltd.
ISBN 978-981-4463-58-4 (Hardcover), 978-981-4463-59-1 (eBook)
www.panstanford.com

value, or expanding land available for agricultural use—all of which can contribute to improved food security. Plants can be used for growing drugs and vaccines. Modern biotechnology has the potential to contribute to poverty alleviation through improvements in health and food security, boosting economic development prospects. In the security realm, biodefense (i.e., defense against biological attack) capabilities can be improved through use of genetic engineering technologies. However, it is extremely unlikely that the revolution will have only positive consequences—historically this has not been the case with any major new technology.

Jeremy Rifkin points this out in *The Biotech Century* (1998):

> If history has taught us anything, it is that every new technological revolution brings with it both benefits and costs. The more powerful the technology is at expropriating and controlling the forces of nature, the more exacting the price we will be forced to pay in terms of disruption and destruction wreaked on the ecosystems and social systems that sustain life. (pp. 35–36)

The negative consequences of the biotechnology revolution may well be severe due to an unprecedented level of directed interference with natural processes. While modern biotechnology can give us new tools to manage environmental problems it also presents new dangers, particularly in its threat to biodiversity. It may also present new threats to human health. It certainly challenges many human values and beliefs. Development may be hampered by changes in ownership patterns in relation to novel crops and seeds and related shifts to monocultural agriculture practices. And the same tools that can improve biodefense can also be used to create more effective biological warfare agents, increasing the threat of their use.

In addition to these more specific consequences, the biotechnology revolution will have more general consequences. Changes in the geography of agricultural production are likely to occur, and changes in global trade relations may create new winners and losers or act to reinforce current inequalities. There will be changes in labor relations and in manufacturing processes. Many ethical dilemmas are raised by the new technologies and the possibilities they bring. People will face new choices about health care and reproduction. Social values and beliefs may have to adjust to incorporate new knowledge. Far more knowledge will be available about people's genetic endowments and what the implications of these are, which also opens the possibility of new forms of discrimination. There are implications for changes in power relations. There will be a need for political direction to deal with many of these challenges while state control is diminishing in areas such as health care.

Significantly the consequences of the biotechnology revolution are unlikely to be evenly spread among nations, and those that are positive for one group may have negative implications for another. Research and development in biotechnology (as in all scientific fields) is overwhelmingly concentrated in rich, developed nations, particularly in the United States, Europe, and Japan. It tends, therefore, to be directed toward meeting the interests of populations in developed nations rather than the needs of the majority of the global population. Current trade and intellectual property laws also favor the interests of the developed countries. Because of this context modern biotechnology may, instead of fulfilling its potential to promote development, exacerbate the gaps between rich and poor, in turn causing increased tensions between the developed and developing worlds. Current global conditions appear to work against the widespread diffusion of innovative technologies and related products to developing countries, preventing the much-needed improvements in health and food security from reaching their populations.

There is a great deal of controversy and debate about exactly what the consequences of modern biotechnology will be. It is impossible to precisely predict the final outcomes of a technological and socioeconomic revolution that is only in its infancy. But there is no doubt that its impacts will be significant, and an examination of debates in the literature gives an indication of their likely scope.

This uncertainty exists largely because there are many factors (beyond the issue of what is technically achievable) that affect the speed and direction of scientific and technological advances in biotechnology and therefore the nature of its applications and their consequences. These include the prevailing political, economic, social, and environmental conditions. Some conditions will drive technological change forward, others will hold it back, and there will be changes in these conditions across time and space, creating a complex interplay that frustrates exact foresight.

Because there are so many potential benefits of these new biotechnologies it is desirable to move forward with the biotechnology revolution. It will at the same time be desirable to avoid the negative consequences of these new technologies. And, because the tensions caused by increased inequalities between rich and poor could impede the development of the biotechnology revolution, and because these gaps hinder full realization of its benefits, it is also desirable to try to spread the benefits as evenly as possible.

Specific Consequences of Biotechnology Applications

Biotechnology has a huge range of applications. So far most developments have been concentrated in the pharmaceutical and agricultural industries. Many claims are made about the positive and negative consequences of applications of modern biotechnology, and the literature in this area is mostly polarized between that which emphasizes costs and that which emphasizes benefits. The products of genetic engineering began to emerge in the markets only in the early 1980s. This means that the long-term consequences of even the earliest commercial applications of modern biotechnology are yet to be fully assessed.

In an attempt to give a more balanced view of potential consequences of some specific biotechnology applications, this essay starts by providing examples of both positive and negative consequences in the areas of environment, health, development* and (protection against) misuse as illustrations of debates in the literature. There is also discussion of the uneven spread of consequences of the biotechnology revolution. The current global context means that the benefits (positive consequences) are likely to be concentrated in the developed world. If this occurs it is likely to influence the direction and speed of the revolution, and it will also create difficulties for the full realization of the revolution's benefits, many of which are claimed on behalf of the poor but may not reach them. Developing countries are also less likely to have the capacity to deal with any negative consequences.

Positive consequences

- **Environmental:** A major aim in the genetic modification of agricultural crops has been to reduce the use of environmentally harmful inputs, creating crops that are cheaper to grow and more environmentally friendly. Use of agricultural chemicals/ biologics (such as pesticides and herbicides) poses a threat to the environment and often to human health as well, and so a reduction in the use of these products will be beneficial. Some of the negative environmental effects of pesticides are listed by Dinham (1993) as "water pollution, soil degradation, insect resistance and resurgence, the destruction of native flora and fauna, and some, as ozone depleters, contribute to the greenhouse effect" (p. 64).

  Two examples of plant genetic engineering for this purpose are the creation of crops that tolerate the application of

---

*When discussed in this essay, development has broader connotations than simply economic growth, referring to other factors that can contribute to the worsening or alleviation of poverty, including food security, health, sanitation, innovative capacities, and modes of ownership.

glyphosate herbicides, such as Roundup Ready™ soybeans, and crops with a Bt gene inserted. Bt stands for *Bacillus thuringiensis*, spores of which, when ingested by certain insects, produce a toxin that kills the insect. The gene transferred to Bt crops is that which codes for production of this toxin. When crops have the Bt gene inserted they gain enhanced resistance to attack by certain pests and the need for applications of insecticide is significantly reduced.

Worldwide in 2009 almost 16.1 million hectares of genetically modified (GM)[†] cotton and 69.2 million hectares of GM soybeans were grown (International Service for the Acquisition of Agri-biotech Applications, 2009). Data from the United States Department of Agriculture's National Agricultural Statistics Service (NASS) indicates a reduction in the use of Bt on cotton and a switch to glyphosate herbicides (from more toxic alternatives) for soybeans since these new crops were introduced. The percentage of cotton acreage treated with Bt in the United States fell from 15% in 1995 to 3% in 2000 (no statistics are provided after 2000), and the percentage of soybean acreage treated with glyphosate rose from 20% in 1995 to 91% in 2006, while at the same time three more toxic alternatives fell in usage from 20% to 2%, from 26% to 3%, and from 44% to 3%, respectively, for trifluralin, pendimethalin, and imazethapyr (NASS, n.d.). However, the Union of Concerned Scientists (UCS) has reported that, after the first few years of planting in the United States, glyphosate-tolerant crops have required increasing amounts of herbicide in comparison to conventional crops as weed resistance has become a significant problem (UCS, 2004, pp. 35–36).

[†]In a discussion of crops that have had their genetic codes manipulated through modern biotechnological techniques, there are three key terms used:
- Genetically engineered (GE): This refers to all crops that have had their genetic codes altered through direct intervention at the genetic level.
- Transgenic: This term refers to those crops that have received genetic information from an unrelated organism.
- Genetically modified (GM): This refers to food products derived from GE crops.

Genetic engineering of crops appears to have been successful in reducing the use of harmful agricultural pesticides, which should have environmental benefits, but it is unclear whether these benefits will persist in the long term.

- **Health:** Advances in genomics (deciphering the genetic codes of living organisms) are providing a greater understanding of diseases, which should lead to the development of better treatments and preventative measures. It is the opinion of the World Health Organisation (WHO) (2002) that "given the huge burden of infectious diseases in developing countries, this research has the potential to change the lives of millions of people." An understanding of individual differences in susceptibility to diseases and in responses to treatments should allow tailoring of drugs to meet individual needs, providing more effective treatment and reducing undesirable side effects.

One disease to which modern biotechnology is being applied is malaria. The genome sequences of the mosquito *Anopheles gambiae* and of the most deadly malarial parasite *Plasmodium falciparum* were both published in October 2002. This information should enable more effective targeting of drugs and increase the understanding of resistance mechanisms so that drugs can be produced to work around them. Projects building on this information[‡] include attempts to eradicate the malarial parasite, to make mosquitoes resistant to the parasite, and to make mosquitoes infertile, as well as creating "new drugs, mosquito-repellents, insecticides and vaccines" (Young, 2002).

According to recent figures published by WHO, malaria caused approximately 247 million cases of acute illness

---

[‡] For details of such work, see, for example, work undertaken at the Malaria Research Institute at Johns Hopkins University (http://www.malaria.jhsph.edu): Marshall, J. M., and Taylor, C. E. (2009). Malaria control with transgenic mosquitoes. *PLoS Medicine*, **6**(2), e.1000020; Webster, D., and Hill, A. V. S. (2003). Progress with new malaria vaccines. *Bulletin of the World Health Organisation*, **81**(12), 902–908; and Cumberland, S. (2009). Mosquito wars. *Bulletin of the World Health Organisation*, **87**, 167–169.

and over 880,000 deaths in 2006 (WHO, 2008a, 2008b) and is estimated to account for up to 40% of public health expenditure in the worst-affected countries (Commission on Sustainable Development, 2006). Clearly finding a means of preventing transmission of this disease will be hugely beneficial. And this is only one of the diseases that modern biotechnology has the potential to help prevent, treat, eradicate, or cure. Additionally, gene therapies (therapies that aim to correct expression of faulty genes) may help combat or prevent genetic diseases such as Huntington's disease, thalassemia, and sickle cell anemia. Modern biotechnology has the potential to bring huge benefits to human health.

- **Development:** Another motivation behind the genetic engineering of crops is to increase yields and improve nutritional value, both of which could make significant contributions to food security. The Food and Agriculture Organization (FAO) states that "food security exists when all people, at all times, have physical and economic access to sufficient, safe and nutritious food to meet their dietary needs and food preferences for an active and healthy life" (FAO, n.d.). The number of undernourished people worldwide passed 1 billion for the first time in 2008 (FAO, 2010). Populations in developed countries account for less than 2% of this figure.

   The above-mentioned engineering of crops for herbicide and pesticide resistance, as well as having positive environmental impacts, should result in a reduction of crop losses and thus increase yield. The nutritional value of crops can be enhanced by inserting genes novel to the plant so that useful additional proteins are produced. A variety of rice known as "Golden Rice" has been created, which contains betacarotene (a precursor to vitamin A). Research on enhanced nutritional value is also underway on rice, sorghum, cassava, and banana under the Grand Challenges in Global Health Programme (n.d.). Micronutrient deficiencies are estimated to account for 1.62 billion cases of anemia, almost 2 billion cases of iodine deficiency (741 million at clinical levels), and 250 million cases of childhood vitamin A deficiency each year (FAO, 2003; WHO, 2008b; WHO, n.d.). The nutritional value of crops used for animal feed can also be enhanced, removing the need for and expense of additives. Food security is not only based on the availability of food, but modern biotechnology also has great potential to improve that aspect of food security.

- **Protection against misuse:** In recent years the threat of attacks using biological weapons has been perceived to increase. Terrorist attacks aimed at causing mass casualties have raised awareness of the possibility of attacks with weapons of mass destruction (biological, chemical, and radiological). Letters containing anthrax sent in late September and October 2001 in the United States demonstrated the widespread fear and disruption that even a low-level, limited-casualty biological attack can have. All of this has led some countries, particularly the United States, to increase their research and development into defense against such attacks. Governmental funding for biodefense in the United States rose from $568 million in 2001 to over $6 billion for 2010, with a high of over $8 billion in 2005 (Franco, 2009).

  Genetic and genomic technologies can be extremely useful in such work against biological attacks, assisting in the creation of detection devices, vaccines, treatments, and countermeasures. The National Institute of Allergy and Infectious Disease (NIAID) *Biodefense Research Agenda for CDC Category A Agents: Responding through Research* released in 2002 "focuses on the need for basic research on the biology of the microbe, the host response and basic and applied research aimed at the development of diagnostics, therapeutics and vaccines against these agents" (NIAID, 2002). The agenda particularly recognizes the significance of genomics in aiding the understanding of human immune responses and susceptibilities to biological agents. Protection against misuse extends beyond biodefense research, including, for example, health-monitoring systems in which genomics can assist in the identification and tracing of disease outbreaks.

Summary

There is clear potential for many, often very important, positive consequences to emerge from the biotechnology revolution. These include improvements to human, animal, and plant health, less environmentally damaging forms of agricultural production, enhanced food security, and new means of defense against biological attacks. This is not the whole story, however, and there are potentially many negative consequences that should not be ignored when considering governance of the revolution.

Negative consequences

- **Environmental:** While the use of genetically engineered (GE) crops may bring environmental benefits through reduced use of agricultural chemicals, there is concern that they also threaten environmental stability. A prominent concern is that cultivation of GE crops will lead to reductions in biodiversity. Biodiversity is essential for environmental stability and is recognized to form an essential resource base, valuable for food security and sustainable development. Indeed, as Madeley (1996) explains, "This diverse variety is an essential link in the food chain—it is the base for increased productivity and it gives humankind the capacity to adapt and develop crops for the future" (p. 6).

  The Convention on Biodiversity Secretariat (2009) defines biodiversity as "the variety of life on Earth, from the simplest bacterial gene to the vast, complex rainforests of the Amazon." GE crops could threaten biodiversity in several ways.

  Current commercial cultivation of GE crops appears to encourage the spread of monocultural farming practices, which reduce the diversity of crops grown. Rather than cultivating a number of different varieties of a particular crop, farmers are encouraged to plant only the specific GE variety. Monocultures are more vulnerable to disease and pests because what affects one plant will affect the entire crop, instead of there being varied resistance (Madeley, 1996, p. 9). Zilberman, Ameden, and Qaim (2007) point out that this is likely to be a particular problem for low-income countries that have "limited capacity to genetically modify local varieties' and so may rely solely on limited range of GE varieties" (p. 73).

GE crops may also threaten biodiversity through effects on other plants both within and across species. GE crops may be advantaged against other wild relatives, pushing them out of ecosystems. There is also the risk of horizontal gene transfer (transfer of the novel genetic trait to other plants), which could result in weeds developing insect resistance or herbicide tolerance. Or the genes may transfer to insects or bacteria, causing them to take up resistance, too. The increased use of glyphosate herbicides on tolerant GE crops has also promoted resistance in weeds (UCS, 2004).

There is additional concern about the direct and indirect effects of GE crops on insects and other wildlife. They may affect and kill untargeted insects directly or have indirect effects on other wildlife, because if insects are eradicated, this has knock-on effects for the rest of the food chain (Rissler and Mellon, 1996, p. 42). Even though farmers may view certain insects as pests, they also form part of larger ecosystems, and the effects of their removal from these systems may be extremely damaging (Pilnick, 2002, p. 129). There is also the potential for toxic proteins to pass up the food chain.

Some examples of contamination via horizontal gene transfer have been found, including a study conducted in October and November of 2000 in which genetic contamination of non-GE varieties of maize was found in Mexico, which is a natural center of maize biodiversity (Quist and Chapela, 2001), and reports of contamination of non-GE oilseed rape in Australia and Japan in August 2005 (ABC News Online, 2005). Insect resistance to the Bt toxin has also been documented in field and laboratory studies but does not appear to be a significant problem for farmers yet (Griffits, Whitacre, Stevens, and Araion, 2001; UCS, 2004); in fact some studies have shown an increase in insect populations where Bt cotton is grown, due to the reduction in use of insecticides (Marvier, McCreedy, Regetz, and Kareiva, 2007; Pray and Naseem, 2007).

A complicating factor is that many of the environmental consequences of the introduction of GE crops are likely to be seen only over the longer term. The Organisation for Economic Co-operation and Development (OECD) recognized this problem in its book *21st Century Technologies: Promises and Perils of a Dynamic Future* (1998):

> Transgenic plants have been on the market only a few years and the effects of cultivation and consumption over a long period are not yet known. It is possible that ecological damage will only occur after ten, twenty or thirty years. (p. 94)

The insects that affect cotton, for example, have historically taken 10 to 15 years to build resistance to new herbicides (UCS, 2004).

- **Health:** While biotechnology has the potential to achieve vast improvements in human health, current side effects to gene therapies have brought its use into question. This may just be a temporary obstacle until further advances are made, but it is a reminder that there is still a lot that is not known about the working of genes, exactly how a living organism reacts to genetic interventions, and that "trying to alter genes without fully understanding their functions could have disastrous consequences" (Pilnick, 2002, p. 108).

An example of problematic side effects can be seen in the case of gene therapy given to several boys suffering from severe combined immunodeficiency disorder (SCID): "Gene therapy in this case involved providing a normal copy of the defective gene which causes SCID, so enabling the normal growth and development of the immune system" (Pilnick, 2002, p. 109).

While the therapy seemed successful in treating the condition, it is also believed to have been responsible for causing leukemia in two of the patients. The reason for the children developing cancer is suggested to be "because the gene inserted next to an oncogene, called Lmo2, in a single white blood cell. This could have triggered the cell to proliferate uncontrollably, causing the disease" (McDowell, 2003).

In addition to problems in controlling the targeting of inserted genetic material, concerns have also been raised about the type of vectors used to carry the material into cells. These are generally modified viruses. The Human Genome Project (HGP) in its information on gene therapy (Department of Energy, 2009) states that the use of viral vectors "present[s] a variety of potential problems to the patient—toxicity, immune and inflammatory response, and gene control and targeting issues. In addition there is always the fear that the viral vector, once inside the patient, may recover its ability to cause disease." Current gene therapies have not involved interventions that can be inherited; concerns are even higher about the effects of gene therapies where the genetic manipulation can be passed on from generation to generation.

Concerns about the health effects of consumption of GM foods have also been voiced. These include concerns that allergens might be transferred along with intended traits or that new allergens could be created and that antibiotic-resistant, or other, genes may transfer to human gut bacteria, resulting in harmful combinations. These concerns are reflected in paragraphs 47 and 51 of the Codex Alimentarius Commission's (CAC) *Guideline for the Conduct of Food Safety Assessment of Foods Produced Using Recombinant-DNA Microorganisms* (2003a):

Genes derived from known allergenic sources should be assumed to encode an allergen and be avoided unless scientific evidence demonstrates otherwise; strains in which antibiotic resistance is encoded by transmissible genetic elements should not be used where such strains or these genetic elements are present in the final food.

Very few long-term assessments of the effects of GM foods on human (or animal) health have been conducted, but in many cases there are unlikely to be additional negative impacts to those of the "conventional counterpart."[§]

- **Development**: While biotechnologies may provide benefits in the area of food security, there may also be negative effects stemming from the way in which they are applied. These could, for example, result from reductions in biodiversity (mentioned above) and also through changes in the patterns of ownership of seeds. Reductions in biodiversity undermine long-term food security because they reduce the available alternatives to currently cultivated crops. Private companies in the United States and Europe develop the vast majority of GM plants and seeds. Because of the costs of research and development these companies feel that it is necessary and justified to protect their inventions through patents and other forms of intellectual property rights. It is the view of the International Chamber of Commerce 2002 that "as with any emerging industry, the protection of intellectual property rights and progressive trade policies are essential to ensure continued innovation and to stimulate investment in biotechnology."

Farmers wishing to use particular GE seeds will, therefore, generally have to buy them from private producers and in many cases will be prohibited from saving seeds from one year to the next and from exchanging seeds with other farmers.

[§]A "conventional counterpart" is in this context defined by the CAC (2003b) as "a related organism/variety, its components and/or products for which there is experience of establishing safety based on common use as food."

Saving of seeds is a widespread and long-standing practice in many developing countries and helps to keep the costs of farming down. Some GE seeds were developed with so-called "terminator technology," which created sterile seeds that could be used for only one season. Due to resistance this technology has not yet been commercially applied.

If farmers are left with little choice but to use corporately owned seeds and plant varieties, at higher cost than traditional sources (such as exchange), this is likely to increase poverty, while pushing out indigenous varieties, leaving little to fall back on. The additional costs of GM seeds may thus be prohibitive, particularly to small-scale farmers in the developing world, meaning that they are unable to use the technology or gain any benefit from it. Indeed, a UCS report points to greater yield increases being achievable by, for example, a switch to organic methods in developing countries than through the use of GE crops (UCS, 2009, p. 5). It is also the case that "the traits that have been introduced in GM crops to date tend to largely favor the existing farming practices of industrial agriculture, rather than meet the needs of the poor" (Pray and Naseem, 2007, p. 193).

- **Misuse**: A greater understanding of diseases and their interactions with humans can result in better treatments, but the same knowledge can be misused, and many of the same technologies and techniques of modern biotechnology that can be applied to enhance defensive capabilities can also be put to hostile use. Several authors (e.g., Dando, 1999; International Committee of the Red Cross [ICRC], 2002; Meselson, 2000; Rifkin, 1998) point to the continuing historical trend for scientific developments to be used for hostile purposes.

   The characteristics of specificity, environmental persistence, infectiousness, and lethality are generally sought in the development of a biological weapon. Genetic engineering technologies have the potential to improve on these aspects, increasing the overall effectiveness of biological weapons, which can only serve to make them more attractive to countries and terrorist groups. The ICRC in its initiative on biotechnology, weapons, and humanity (launched in 2002) identifies eight main concerns regarding the use of biotechnology in the production of biowarfare agents. These are (ICRC, 2002):

1. Manipulation of known biological warfare agents
2. Harmless microbes being made dangerous
3. Development of hostile vaccinations
4. Research that may lead to unintended but dangerous outcomes
5. Artificial creation of extremely dangerous viruses
6. Undetected attacks that can alter bodily functions
7. "Genetic weapons"
8. Effects on agriculture and infrastructure

Point 7 of this list relates to the fear that future genetic engineering technology may be able to create biological agents that can target specific groups of people. This possibility increases as genomic knowledge of humans and of disease-causing microorganisms expands. Much of this knowledge is being placed in the public domain. The genomes of several disease-causing microbes—including, controversially, the 1918 influenza virus—have already been sequenced and published, and research is underway on establishing the genetic differences between groups that account for different susceptibilities to disease. This work is being carried out inter alia in the Haplotype Map Project of the US National Genome Research Institute. Its website states that "the haplotype map, or 'HapMap,' is a tool that allows researchers to find genes and genetic variations that affect health and disease" (National Human Genome Research Institute, 2009).

The uneven spread of consequences

The biotechnology revolution brings negative consequences alongside positive ones. Equally problematic is the fact that these consequences will not be evenly distributed among countries. If the biotechnology revolution serves to widen the gap between rich and poor this will be a significant negative consequence in itself. This effect of the biotechnology revolution is a result of the global context in which the revolution is occurring rather than being inherent to the technology.

The biotechnology revolution is taking place in an increasingly globalized world, and it is a global phenomenon in terms of its effects. This globalized world is one of great inequalities, dominated by the economic power of a few developed countries. This context is an important factor that influences how the impacts of modern biotechnology will be spread. Particularly, current trends mean that developed countries will benefit more than developing countries, due to their much larger capacities for research and development, their dominance of international markets, and their more advanced regulatory systems. Developed countries are also likely to have greater capacities to cope with socioeconomic change and to deal with the negative effects of the new technologies.

Research and development in the health care sector is disproportionately concentrated in the developed world, with an estimated 90% of research and development taking place there (where approximately 20% of the world's population lives). Pharmaceutical research and development is a very costly and time-consuming process, so companies seek to recoup their money by protecting their inventions and selling their drugs generally at higher rates than the cost price. Few people or governments in the developing world can afford these prices. This means that pharmaceutical companies have little incentive to produce drugs and vaccines to meet the developing world's needs (such as combating tropical diseases), so most research and development is done to meet the needs of people in the developed world. As Goonatilake (1999, p. 120) points out, the same is true for biotechnology-based pharmaceuticals: "Market forces thus determine what is considered a commercially desirable biotechnology product. Operating globally these forces preselect particular biological products for research, development and production."

Ill health contributes to poverty and constrains development. Gaps in health are therefore closely related to the gap between rich and poor and contribute to it. Clearly, as Qaim (2000, p. 8) argues, "If biotechnology R&D would only benefit the richer population segments while neglecting the needs of the poor, the innovation could engender an aggravation of existing income disparities." Differences in regulatory capacity in the health area are also of concern to WHO (2002), which pointed out in *Genomics and World Health: Report of the Advisory Committee on Health Research* that "a general feature of many developing countries is a lack of well-developed regulatory apparatus to deal with either the scientific issues in genetic research and technology, or with the ethical, legal and social issues." Countries may also lack necessary experience and expertise for timely and effective policy making in these areas.

This concentration of benefits in the developed world may well exacerbate gaps between rich and poor; it may also cause tensions between countries and contribute to resistance to the new technologies. Examples of this have already been seen in campaigns by developing countries against patents on drugs and resistance to food aid that contains GM products. These issues have caused tensions in international forums, particularly in the World Trade Organization (WTO) because of its agreement that requires harmonization of national patent rules (the Agreement on Trade Related Aspects of Intellectual Property Rights, or TRIPS).

At a meeting of the WTO in Doha in 2001, developing countries challenged the patent rights held by and licensing practices of multinational pharmaceutical companies and the resulting costs of essential medicines. This campaign was partially successful and is ongoing. The November 2001 *Doha Declaration* of the WTO (2001) states in paragraph 17:

> We stress the importance we attach to implementation and interpretation of the Agreement on Trade Related Aspects of Intellectual Property Rights (TRIPS Agreement) in a manner supportive of public health, by promoting both access to essential medicines and research and development into new medicines and, in this connection, are adopting a separate declaration."

The separate declaration was the *Declaration on the TRIPS Agreement and Public Health*, under which developing countries would be allowed to "seek a waiver on public health grounds from strict WTO rules which guarantee drug patents for 20 years" (Denny, 2001). However, some countries, particularly the United States, refused to support the declaration, so it has had little practical effect (BBC News Online, 2002).

Some developing countries seem particularly wary of, and have opposed, having products of agricultural biotechnology forced upon them, before concerns about their safety for health and the environment have been answered, particularly when the products have not been designed with their needs in mind and when they are unsure what it will mean in terms of export markets. In autumn 2002 while parts of its population faced starvation, Zambia refused to accept food aid that contained GM products. Other African countries (Malawi, Mozambique, Lesotho, and Zimbabwe) insisted that such food aid be milled before distribution so that farmers could not use the seeds (Knight, 2002). Again, due to market forces, research and development in this area is concentrated on the needs of farmers in the developed world. Most developments have been for crops grown in the United States (predominantly soybean, maize, canola, and cotton) and suited to defeating the pests and diseases prevalent there and to growth in particular environmental conditions. Pray and Naseem (2007, pp. 193–194) outline some of the main forces at work here:

- Multinational firms are unwilling to make necessary investments in biotechnology research relevant to developing country agriculture due to limited market potential, fear of piracy of their intellectual property, and the high cost of meeting regulatory requirements. Taken together, this has meant that research on crops important to poor farmers yields low private returns and hence provides limited incentives for private firms to invest.
- Development of new crops aimed at meeting the needs of farmers in the developing world has been largely left to small, public research centers. Developing countries generally lack the capacity to undertake much basic research—although there are some exceptions to this, such as India and China— and these countries may also lack "the scientific capacity to know which technologies would be most useful, or how to use them even if they were to get access" (Pray and Naseem, 2007). Additionally many developing countries lack regulatory and risk assessment capacities supportive of safe development and application of these technologies (Thies and Devare, 2007).
- The environmental risks from GE crops will be highest in areas that are centers of biodiversity, which are concentrated in the developing world, because gene transfers are more likely to occur where the engineered crop is in close proximity to wild relatives. Also the costs of containment and cleanup of environmental damage may well be unaffordable to many developing nations. This means that the countries that are most likely to be negatively affected by the biotechnology revolution will probably be those that are also least able to cope with these effects.

Summary

Due to the international context, while the impacts of the biotechnology revolution are and will continue to be globally felt they are not evenly distributed. Private companies based in the developed world dominate research and development for many applications of biotechnology, and the products of biotechnology are focused on the needs of their populations. Such uneven distribution of the consequences of modern biotechnology seems likely to further widen existing gaps between rich and poor within and between the developing and developed worlds. In turn this will cause tensions that could impede the progress of the biotechnology revolution. Most importantly it is likely to prevent the much-needed advances in food security and health becoming a reality for the world's poor.

Specific consequences: Conclusion

When looking at the consequences of specific applications of biotechnology, although precise outcomes may be unclear, there are still some obvious trends that can be identified. There will be both positive and negative impacts arising from the biotechnology revolution. Evidence of impacts is limited so far as the revolution remains in its infancy, and many effects are likely to appear only over the long term. This is the view of the OECD (1998):

> Since modern biotechnology goes back only a few decades, its possibilities are by no means exhausted, although it is difficult to assess their range and impact. Modern biotechnology is therefore a scientific and technological development trend which is at the beginning of its life cycle. (p. 77)

Modern biotechnology has the potential to greatly improve human health but also presents it with new hazards. It has the potential to reduce and counter humanity's negative impacts on the environment but also to cause devastating loss of biodiversity. It has the potential to help feed the world, but it may also result in greater food insecurity. It can create better defense against biological attack but also encourage and enable development of improved biological weapons. Finally, the consequences will be different for different countries. The claimed benefits biotechnology will bring to the poor may not reach them. The benefits could well remain concentrated in the developed world.

General Consequences of the Biotechnology Revolution

Alongside the specific consequences associated with particular applications of modern biotechnology, there will be many, more general socioeconomic consequences. Again, most of these consequences will be felt globally and their impacts will vary between nations. Something that is (perceived as) positive for one country or group may be (perceived as) negative for another. These more general consequences are not yet widely seen, and indeed many may be hard to quantify; however, their effects are likely to be substantial.

Prentis (1984), in *Biotechnology: A New Industrial Revolution*, explains that all major technological change has socioeconomic consequences and that the biotechnology revolution will be no exception:

> Any major new technology has profound social, economic and political effects. Biotechnology is no exception, and the potential consequences of the growth of biotechnological industries on the health of workers and on the public, on national and international trade, on economic power and on the position of science in society need to be examined. (p. 171)

Because the changes involved deeply impact life processes themselves, societies will face challenges to values and beliefs about life. Genetic interventions raise many ethical dilemmas, which societies and governments must struggle with. Genomics will produce new forms of knowledge, which will present novel choices in health and reproduction but could also provide the basis of additional forms of discrimination. The OECD (1998, p. 41) argues that "no aspect of the human being, whether physical, mental, intellectual, social, psychological or physiological, will be beyond practical manipulation and change, all of which will be made possible and practical through technology."

In the economic realm there are likely to be changes in patterns of international trade, changes in the geography of (agricultural) production, new economic winners and losers and new labor relations, and changes in production processes. These socioeconomic effects may also bring about political changes. Particularly there may be a need to enable democratic debates to take place to resolve ethical dilemmas and to facilitate choice making. New forms of state control may be demanded (e.g., to prevent genetic discrimination or limit genetic interventions), while at the same time some areas that are now dominated by the state may move to more individual control (e.g., health care options). It is Yoxen's (1986, p. 212) view of the biotechnology revolution that "it is a major economic phenomenon that will have social and political repercussions. It will affect the patterns of trade . . . it will force some industries to the wall, it will have profound effects on the global structures of power."

Of course there are many factors that will influence exactly what happens, and capacities to deal with such changes vary, but it is clear that modern biotechnology will result in significant and widespread socioeconomic change.

Economic changes

The new biotechnologies have rapidly found commercial application. The raw materials used in research and development and the resulting products are traded on international markets. Often they present an alternative or substitute for current products and as such can result in major shifts in demand. This could cause significant changes in trade relations, but it may also strengthen current trends in the dominance of international trade by a few rich nations and multinational companies.

Changes in the geography of agricultural production could occur if countries decide to adapt a crop (like coffee) that they currently import so as to grow successfully in their local climate. This is a possibility because, as Bijman, van den Doel, and Junne (1987, p. 3) explain, "Biotechnology has meant that plants which could only be grown in a certain area for climatic reasons can now be grown elsewhere, thus representing new competition for the traditional producers."

The biotechnology revolution will also bring changes to production in other industries, particularly those based on petrochemicals and those involved in the processing of food. Goonatilake (1999, p. 134) explains what changes in trade could mean for developing countries: "The change will signify a lesser use of earlier raw materials and so a weakening of the trade links established in the 19th century. The effect on commodity exports from the developing world because of biotechnology would therefore be dramatic."

Technological revolutions also cause changes in labor relations. Biotechnology will probably reinforce trends toward knowledge-based economies in the developed world since many of its applications emerge directly from basic research. In the developing world labor changes are more likely to result from changes in agricultural production as many GE crops suit large-scale, industrialized farming methods.

Social implications of human genetics

All major technological change has social impacts. Those associated with modern biotechnology are potentially huge because of the unprecedented level of control over and the ability to intervene in basic life processes involved. The social impacts will be many, varied, and complex. The exact impacts will, of course, vary between societies, but because of the global nature of the biotechnology revolution, it is likely to impact in some way on the vast majority of societies. Many of the most direct social impacts are emerging from advances in human genetics. A few of the major concerns about the social impacts of modern biotechnology will be outlined here— including possible eugenic outcomes, discrimination, and new social divisions—but first a brief overview of advances in human genetics is provided.

Developments in human genetics

Advances in human genetics have centered on two main areas: genomics, which has provided and continues to provide new knowledge and understanding of the human genome, the functions of certain genes, and their interaction with diseases and environmental influences, and genetic engineering, which provides the tools to apply this knowledge, most successfully at present through genetic testing and screening, but also in the form of gene therapy.

Genomics is the study of genomes, that is, the complete genetic sequences of organisms. Significant advances in the study of the human genome have taken place in the international, publicly funded HGP and its private rival Celera, both of which published draft sequences of the human genome in February 2001. The final draft of the human genome was announced in April 2003. The HGP is now concentrating on discovering and mapping the functions of genes and on understanding how they interact with each other and with external factors. A particular purpose of human genomics is to facilitate understanding of disease mechanisms and genetic disorders and to identify the particular genes involved so that they can be targeted for treatment. Pharmacogenomics, a subdiscipline of genomics, is the study of how genes interact with certain pharmaceutical drugs. This work is done to improve the effectiveness of drugs, avoid adverse reactions, and minimize side effects. This has the potential to lead to "tailor made" drug treatments designed to be safe and optimally effective for a particular individual's physiological responses.

New knowledge of human genes and their role in disease is already being applied through genetic screening, testing, and gene therapy. The terms "genetic screening" and "genetic testing" are often used interchangeably, although they can be differentiated with genetic screening applying to whole population groups and genetic testing applying to individuals. Genetic testing is carried out to find out whether "abnormal" genes or harmful genetic mutations are present and is done to test the individual for a particular disease/disorder, for the risk of developing a particular disease, or for the risk of carrying a gene for a hereditary disorder. Genetic testing can be carried out on fetuses in the first few months of pregnancy, giving the option of termination if the fetus is shown to be carrying a mutation. More recently there has emerged the possibility of testing embryos in vitro and selecting only "healthy" embryos to be implanted. This technique is known as preimplantation genetic diagnosis (PGD).

Once a gene has been identified as having a fault that makes it responsible for causing a disease or disorder, and it has been located on the genome, then there is the possibility (at least for single-gene genetic disorders) of intervention to correct that fault. This can be done through the provision of "correct" copies of the gene transmitted, usually through a viral vector, into the cells of the patient. This is known as gene therapy. While gene therapy has had little success so far and has run into some problems, there is still a lot of research being conducted in this area, and it will probably have more widespread application in the future. Gene therapy is, so far, being limited to interventions in somatic cells (e.g., cells that are not involved in reproduction) so that the genetic changes cannot be inherited.

Concerns about possible eugenic outcomes

One concern that is frequently raised is that new genetic knowledge and technologies will be used for eugenic purposes. The literal meaning of "eugenic" is "good gene." The idea behind eugenics is the improvement of the human gene pool by promoting the inheritance of "good" genes (known as positive eugenics) and removing "bad" genes from the gene pool (known as negative eugenics). Eugenic practices have a long but generally troubled history having been used to justify genocide and human rights abuses. The ability of new genetic technologies to be put to eugenic uses has raised alarm over a potential return to past abuses. Appleyard (1999) outlines the reasons for such concern:

> Precisely because a belief in fundamental biological differences has led to such horrors in the past, and precisely because it is obvious that such knowledge was deliberately rigged to provide a spurious basis for bigotry, we should be very, very, cautious about using biological differences to explain behavior, personality or even disease. The history of biological justifications is a bloody one, far too bloody for us ever to contemplate taking such risks again. (p. 47)

This is an extremely complicated issue; there are different types of eugenics and not all are perceived (by everyone) as bad. Societies face the problem of deciding where and how to draw the line when it comes to selecting "good" genes over "bad" genes. That sort of selection is already implicit in genetic testing, screening, and therapy, where there is always some notion of a "faulty" or "abnormal" gene involved. Indeed Rifkin (1998) raises the point that all genetic engineering decisions are inherently eugenic choices involving the selection of one gene over another:

> Every time a genetic change of this kind is made, the scientist, corporation or state is implicitly, if not explicitly, making

a decision about which are the good genes that should be inserted and preserved and which are the bad genes that should be altered or deleted. (p. 128)

Current proponents of eugenics differentiate between past compulsory and enforced state-run eugenics programs and the current opportunity to have voluntary eugenics based on individual choice. However, the idea of voluntary eugenics is also problematic if you recognize that society can exert a great deal of influence over individual choices and that lack of or misinformation about the meaning of test results and the quality of life of individuals suffering from certain diseases may also skew decisions. Several authors (e.g., Appleyard, 1999; Hindmarsh, Lawrence, and Norton, 1998; Pilnick, 2002) raise the point that many individual choices may have the cumulative effect of a national eugenics practice. In the words of Hindmarsh, Lawrence, and Norton (1998, p. 102), "One person's personal preference—when part of a broader trend involving many people—creates the injustice of discrimination against a whole class or category of other people."

It is also necessary to look at the implications that determining certain traits (disease causing or otherwise) as undesirable may have for people already living with those traits. What happens to their right to life? Will they feel fully valued by society? And will the country provide the social services necessary for them to take part in society? WHO (2002), in its report *Genomics and World Health: Report of the Advisory Committee on Health Research*, explains why many disabled people object to prenatal genetic testing: "Disabled people see society's message in supporting genetic testing for the conditions they have as being that it would have been better if they had never been born, a message that they and others quite understandably reject."

If we accept that genetic selection may be permissible under certain circumstances and for certain purposes (e.g., the provision of a stem-cell donor match for a seriously ill sibling) difficulties still arise over what should count as a genetic "fault" that may be corrected, who gets to decide this, and what the implications of this decision will be. While current uses of PGD and prenatal genetic screening have so far mainly been limited to avoiding serious genetic diseases or helping to save the life of an existing child, exactly the same techniques could be used to select embryos on the basis of a whole range of other traits, some of which have nothing to do with disease or impairment, such as sex or eye color. Appleyard (1999) argues that this technology could in the future be used to create "designer" babies:

> More rapid DNA sequencing techniques and greater knowledge about the effects of specific genes would mean that a much larger range of conditions could be sought in the embryonic cell. These conditions need not be what we now classify as serious diseases. In time they could, for example, forecast anything from the eye color, to the likely intelligence or sexual orientation of the child. PGD could offer, to those who could afford it, a choice of what kind of child they would like. (p. 18)

If further research identifies such genes (and it seems likely that it will), selection could take place on the basis of intelligence or behavioral traits. There is even disagreement over what should count as a serious disease. The British Human Genetics Commission (HGC), in its *Debating the Ethical Future of Human Genetics: First Annual Report of the Human Genetics Commission*, advised that "PGD should be limited to specific and serious conditions," while at the same time stating that "it has proved impossible to define what "serious" should mean in this context" (HGC, 2001, pp. 45–46).

Since eugenics labels (implicitly or explicitly) particular traits as normal/abnormal, good/bad, or desirable/undesirable it carries with it an implied relationship of superiority and inferiority between people, which may well undermine the fundamental concept of humans being equal and worthy of equal respect, treatment, and rights. Appleyard (1999) draws attention to the dangers of this:

> The point is that once people decide you are a lesser creature, for whatever reason, either superstitious or scientific, there appears to be no limit to what cruelty they may inflict on you. And they are likely to inflict that cruelty feeling justified, because it is but a small step from believing another human being is inferior to believing that he is bad, dangerous or threatening to "superior" beings. (p. 49)

Concerns about discrimination

New genetic knowledge will provide opportunities for new forms of discrimination. If it is discovered that a particular gene makes someone susceptible to a particular disease, and that gene can be tested for, then insurers and employers (among others) may wish to discriminate on the basis of the presence of the gene in an individual's genome, whether the disease actually develops or it doesn't. Insurance premiums may be set higher or cover refused for individuals carrying certain genes. An example of this is a British woman who found herself unable to get insurance due to carrying the *BRCA2* gene, which has been implicated in some cancers (Boseley, 2003). However, for the moment, most insurers have placed a moratorium on the use of genetic test results. Employers may wish to avoid later litigation if a potential employee is found to have a gene that interacts with the particular working environment to cause a disease.

If genes are found that affect intelligence this may exclude certain people from mainstream schooling. A gene for a behavioral trait like aggression may lead to the refusal to employ someone, as could a gene for mental illness or a propensity to alcoholism. This is despite the fact that such traits are largely socially defined/constructed. Hindmarsh, Lawrence, and Norton (1998, p. 101) state that "a real danger therefore exists that a focus upon genetic factors will result in some people being classified in a manner which excludes them from employment, from education, from access to credit and other financial services, and even from being able to marry and form a family." They also point out that "significantly, a person who is denied access may often not become ill or incapacitated and might never be so" (1998, p. 101).

This same genetic knowledge may well be, in medical terms, extremely beneficial to the individual, allowing early diagnosis, prevention, or treatment of disease. For medical purposes some governments are encouraging the collection of individual genetic information. For example, the UK Department of Health (2003) stated in its genetics white paper that it would consider whether to collect genetic blueprints from all babies at birth. However, societies need to decide who should have access to the information and what it should be used for. There is also a need to consider that an individual may not want to have this information (and may not want the doctor to have it either)—will he or she be given a choice? This is a real possibility. At present some people who may have Huntington's disease choose not to be tested for it, because they do not want to know if they have it, since it cannot be treated. Also what would happen if an individual refuses to act on the genetic information by, for example, refusing to follow dietary and lifestyle advice despite being shown to have an increased risk of heart disease—would he or she be refused state-funded health care/private health insurance?

New genetic knowledge is expected to revolutionize health care and may be very beneficial to society, but it carries many pitfalls and raises new and difficult dilemmas. It is also open to abuse and challenges ideas of privacy, confidentiality, and informed consent.

Changes to values and concepts

The sanctity of life, particularly human life, is a powerful, fundamental, and widely held concept and not just for religious reasons. It is a central concept of many, if not all, societies, and the "right to life" is seen as a basic and core human right (Article 3, Universal Declaration of Human Rights, 1948). Modern genetics and genomic technologies challenge some widely held ideas about life as they allow basic life processes to be manipulated and exploited in a deliberate manner. The right to patent genes (including human genes) is seen by many as an unwanted and unwarranted commodification of life. Genomics can reduce "life" to a code, a form of information, open to intervention and "improvement" by human hands. Appleyard (1999) explains what effect this might have:

> There is no sanctity attached to the individual; rather he or she becomes a collection of characteristics, each of which can be judged on some scale of relative significance. At this point it becomes difficult to distinguish human beings from consumer goods. (p. 134)

Many people thus view genetic technologies and particularly human genetics as fundamentally wrong.

There are also right-to-life issues raised by the use of prenatal genetic testing and PGD, where the former often has abortion as the only alternative and the latter often entails the disposal of several embryos. Similarly there have been objections raised to the use of embryonic stem cells in research, where they have a huge potential to assist in therapies. Research using embryonic stem cells is banned in many countries at present due to moral and ethical objections. PGD is, however, allowed under certain circumstances, and prenatal genetic testing is now routine in many countries.

There are further problems raised by modern biotechnology for concepts of human rights and human responsibilities. What does the concept of a right to health now entail? Does it include the right to have genetic faults corrected? The right to a dignified life is also challenged—what does it mean for someone's dignity if his or her birth is selected on the basis that he or she would save the life of another? Further problems arise if genes are found that influence human behavior—what does this mean for human autonomy and the concept of responsibility for one's own behavior? If it is someone's genes that are the reason for his or her aggression and violence, is it the person's fault if he or she murders someone? Is he or she less culpable? Could he or she have avoided the particular route taken? Should a different term of punishment be applied to such individuals? The example of a gene for aggression is used by Pilnick (2002):

> Raising the question of what societies might practically do with this knowledge poses some uncomfortable answers. If aggression is linked to genetics alone, aggressive behavior may be condoned or seen as inevitable. The principle of the individual's responsibility for their own behavior is undermined. (p. 41)

New genetic technologies are also redefining the social meaning of concepts such as health and sickness, disease, and abnormality. The concept of health is widened beyond being free of symptoms to being free of genetic defects and perhaps even not having the propensity to suffer from certain diseases. Since every individual will have some "faults" in his or her genome, does this then mean that everyone is ill? Some believe that such changes may reduce discrimination, since if everyone carries abnormalities, then this will be perceived as "normal": "Molecular biologists argue that, because the genetic tests they are developing will show that all of us are flawed in one way or another, these tests will bring an end to genetic discrimination" (Hubbard and Wald, 1993, p. 36).

But what will it mean for people to view themselves as unhealthy when there is nothing that can be done? Or to be prescribed life-long treatment for a disease that may never afflict them? This is likely to affect the provision of social services (particularly health care). There is also a fear that this focus on genetics as a cause of disease will lead to environmental factors being ignored and yet, basic sanitation, clean water and improved nutrition could save millions of lives each year (UNICEF, no date) and can be achieved at relatively low cost via application of existing technologies.

Concerns about power and control

Many of the concerns about the social implications of modern biotechnology stem from issues of power and control. Who will make the decisions? Who will have access to the information? And how will they be able/permitted to use it?

Social divisions may widen if access to the benefits of the new technologies is uneven. Kitcher (1996, p. 198) raises the prospect of a future where the rich can afford to pay to have genetically guaranteed healthy and intelligent children, while the poor cannot and find that resources have been diverted from social services and national health care to genetic technologies that benefit the few. New social divisions that occur along genetic lines are feared, particularly if some form of eugenics goes ahead. Hubbard and Wald (1993, p. 36) also point out that discrimination is more likely to affect the already disadvantaged: "Like other forms of discrimination, genetic discrimination will be felt most by people who are already stigmatized in other ways. People with access to power and resources are more likely to be shielded."

Summary

Advances in modern biotechnology have many social implications, although it is difficult to be certain of what the precise effects might be. The new technologies make possible a new form of eugenics, they may encourage genetic discrimination, and they challenge core concepts such as the meaning of life, health, and normality. They may create new social divisions and/or exacerbate existing ones and create tensions and clashes of values. And these advances could undermine the ideals of basic human rights, shared by all. Appleyard (1999, p. 3) provides a good summary point: "Genetics is . . . a historically unique combination of philosophy, science and technology that confronts humanity with the most fundamental questions, our answers to which will determine the human future."

Like the other impacts of modern biotechnology, the social impacts will be global, but not evenly spread, and some societies are likely to have greater capacities to cope with social change and to diffuse any resulting tensions. While countries may choose to prohibit certain uses of the new technologies to protect their social values, the global nature of the biotechnology revolution presents problems for this—research and application of the new technologies can simply move elsewhere. This means that a global response is required.

Political impacts

The political impacts of the biotechnology revolution are closely connected to the nature of its economic and social impacts. Governments are likely to find themselves called upon to take a lead on certain issues, while at the same time finding that their control over certain policy areas is diminishing (with, for example, the individualization and privatization of health care). There is also likely to be demand for greater democratic involvement in policy making on genetics issues and a demand for accountability and transparency in decision making. As the Centre for Genetics Education (2002) states, "Society and its governments will need to consider the boundaries that have to be put in place to monitor developments and ensure ethical applications of this new and advancing technology." Governments will need to formulate policies nationally to deal with the socioeconomic effects of biotechnology and also make an effort to harmonize such policies internationally in order to gain effective control.

General consequences: Conclusion

The biotechnology revolution will result in significant socioeconomic changes. These general consequences of the biotechnology revolution will involve changes in production and employment and in international trade. Many ethical dilemmas have already been raised by the new power over life that genetic technologies bring. Changes in values are likely to occur as the meaning and sanctity of life are challenged. Societies will be presented with new choices and may demand a chance to participate in decisions about the control of these new technologies. New types of discrimination may arise. The overall consequences of these changes may be positive or negative; either way they will result in disruption.

Because the biotechnology revolution is a global phenomenon these socioeconomic changes will occur globally, but the precise nature of their impacts will vary, and negative consequences are more likely to be felt by countries and societies that lack the capacity to deal with such changes. Just as with specific consequences there is uncertainty about what the general consequences of modern biotechnology will be. This is because there are a number of complicating factors that will affect what the exact outcomes of the revolution will be.

Factors Affecting the Speed and Direction of Technological Change and Its Socioeconomic Consequences

It is impossible to predict the precise outcomes of the biotechnology revolution. Certainty is made impossible because of the many complicating factors that can influence the speed and direction of technological change. These include regulatory frameworks, economic conditions, government policies, public perceptions, the cost of alternatives, and environmental necessity. Some of these factors will drive technological change, while others will constrain it. Their influence will vary across space and time. In their report on the global technology revolution, Anton, Silberglitt, and Schneider (2001) explain that "the actual realization of these possibilities will depend on a number of factors, including local acceptance of technological change, levels of technology and infrastructure investment, market drivers and limitations, and technology breakthroughs and advancements. Since these factors will vary across the globe, the implementation effects of technology will also vary, especially in developing countries."

The effects of regulation

Regulation can both drive and impede technological change; it can also influence its course. This is true of national, regional, and international regulation. Because biotechnology has so many different applications a wide range of laws are applicable to it. This means that the revolution is influenced by a variety of standards, guidelines, laws, and conventions, which work in different ways to shape its pace and direction. The various regulations frequently overlap, interact, and compete with each other. Their influence will vary for different applications of biotechnology, between countries and regions, and across time.

Economic conditions

The pace and course of the biotechnology revolution will also be influenced by a variety of economic conditions at various levels—national, regional, and international. The OECD in its 1998 assessment (*21st Century Technologies: Promises and Perils of a Dynamic Future*) considered economic policies that provide a stable economic environment to encourage innovation.

It also stated that "more flexible labour markets, transparent and open capital markets, and competitive goods and services markets are all essential to the fluid resource reallocation and experimentation that is likely to be typical of robust socio-technical dynamism" (p. 31). Conversely, economic recession is likely to slow technological change by discouraging risk taking. International economic conditions and policies such as free trade may encourage innovation by ensuring open markets for end products. Encouragement of competition at any level is also thought to drive technological change by providing an incentive to stay ahead of competitors. The influences created by economic conditions will again vary over time and between countries.

Government policies

In connection with the earlier sections, government regulatory and economic policies will have an influence on the pace and direction of the biotechnology revolution. For example, if a government decides to raise environmental standards this could encourage a move toward alternative energy sources (from fossil fuels to biomass, for example) and to less polluting means of production, which could drive technological change as new alternatives are sought.

An example of government policy that might impede technological change is the decision of some governments to restrict commercial growing of GE crops, which clearly removes a major incentive to develop and market such products. Government policies obviously vary among countries, although there may be some regional harmonization and the policies of international organizations may also have a harmonizing influence; policies also vary over time. Therefore, the influence of policies on the speed and direction of the biotechnology revolution will vary over time and between countries. There are also numerous factors that contribute to the creation and choice of particular policies.

Public views

Where the public resists new technology, at any level from local to global, this can impede technological change or change its course. Public resistance also varies within and between countries and over time. An example of this is public resistance to consumption of GM foods. This resistance has been far more prevalent in Europe than in the United States; these differences are reflected in official policies.

Public resistance often occurs when values are challenged; this can be seen in the area of human cloning, where public responses also vary. While some people reject all human cloning as an affront to human dignity, others view cloning limited to the production of embryonic stem cells for therapeutic uses to be justified under the human right to health. Technological development in the area of therapeutic human cloning has been impeded by government prohibitions in many countries driven by public resistance.

Resistance may change over time as further knowledge of the health and safety implications is gained and as new technological breakthroughs are made, improving the safety of certain procedures or products. Public resistance varies with different applications of biotechnology and sometimes within applications, too.

Costs of alternatives

The potential for new biotechnology products and processes to replace existing ones based on, for example, petrochemicals means that the relative costs of the two alternatives would be a factor affecting the speed of technological change. While petrochemicals remain cheaper than the biotechnology-based alternative, even if there are environmental benefits to be gained by switching products, this is unlikely to happen. For example, while fuel alcohol can be produced from biomass and is considered (at least by some) to be a less polluting alternative, most vehicles still use petrol because fuel alcohol is relatively expensive. This factor also varies across place and time. Brazil makes widespread use of biomass-derived fuel alcohol because in its particular national context it is a cost-effective alternative. So the progress of the biotechnology revolution will also be influenced by the costs of alternative products, processes, and technologies.

Environmental necessity

Environmental necessity may also influence the speed and direction of the biotechnology revolution. Because biotechnology can provide less environmentally damaging alternatives to current energy sources and manufacturing processes, the biotechnology revolution may be driven forward by the necessity to implement such alternatives to reduce pollution. Awareness of the damage humanity is causing to our environment and of our dependence on the planet's life systems is growing and the necessity to act is gaining recognition. This can be seen in the growth of international environmental agreements, such as the Kyoto Protocol, in which governments promised to meet targets in the reduction of greenhouse gas emissions. Modern biotechnology can provide tools and products to help meet such targets.

Summary

One of the reasons for there being such uncertainty about the consequences of the biotechnology revolution is that there are a number of complicating factors that will influence its speed and direction, some of which were discussed above. They include regulatory, economic, and political conditions; public opinion; and environmental necessity. These influences will vary across space and time and can both drive and impede technological change. The nature of these influences and their complex interactions with other factors make them impossible to predict, which means that we cannot be sure of the speed and direction of the biotechnology revolution and its consequences.

Conclusion

Considerable uncertainty remains about precisely what the outcomes of the biotechnology revolution will be. This is partly because the revolution is still in its infancy, with many scientific and technological advances still to come, and because of a lack of information about the long-term effects of even its current applications. The uncertainty is also caused by the unprecedented level of interference in and control over nature that this revolution involves, allowing rapid and direct intervention in the basic processes of life itself. Further significant causes of uncertainty are the complex and unpredictable effects of a wide range of factors that will influence the speed and direction of change.

Despite this uncertainty, some broad points are clear. The biotechnology revolution will bring many positive consequences (or benefits) for human, animal, and plant health, for the environment, for food security and other aspects of development, and for security. The revolution will also have negative consequences in the same areas, threatening health, environmental stability, development, and security. It will also result in general socioeconomic changes and some significant political effects. These broader changes will also have positive and negative aspects.

The biotechnology revolution is occurring within a global context that already includes great disparities in wealth within and between countries and international relations of dominance and dependence socially, economically, and politically. This context means that the consequences of the biotechnology revolution will not be evenly spread. It is likely that the positive consequences will be concentrated in the developed world, which also has a better capacity for dealing with many of the negative consequences. This disparity may well be problematic and not just on humanitarian grounds, particularly if it exacerbates the gap between rich and poor, which is a likely consequence. This may also lead to increased tensions between developed and developing countries and may negatively affect the progress of the revolution by creating resistance to its products.

So while we cannot be certain of the exact outcomes of this revolution, the consequences are potentially huge (both positive and negative). There is a need to decide what is desirable (what applications and what outcomes) and to open up debates on this. There is a need to find mechanisms for coping with the socioeconomic impacts so that change is as smooth and beneficial as possible. The benefits of biotechnology need to be promoted, but at the same time the negative consequences and disruptions need to be minimized. There need to be reductions in the inequalities of benefit distribution, and misuse must be prevented.

References

ABC News Online (2005, 26 August). *Grains Industry to Probe GM Canola Contamination*, http://www.abc.net.au/news/australia/vic/mildura/200508/s1446920.htm (accessed October 15, 2009).

Anton, P. S., Silberglitt, R., and Schneider, J. (2001). *The Global Technology Revolution: Bio/Nano/Materials Trends and Their Synergies with Information Technology by 2015*. RAND/National Defense Research Institute, http://www.rand.org/pubs/monograph_reports/MR1307/index.html (accessed March 31, 2003).

Appleyard, B. (1999). *Brave New Worlds: Genetics and the Human Experience*. London: Harper Collins.

BBC News Online (2002, 21 December). *Trade Rules and Cheap Drugs*, http://news.bbc.co.uk/1/hi/health/1644946.stm (accessed June 4, 2004).

Bijman, J., van den Doel, K., and Junne, G. (1987). *The International Dimension of Biotechnology in Agriculture*. Dublin: European Foundation for the Improvement of Living and Working Conditions.

Boseley, S. (2003, 24 June). It makes me mad that I can't get insurance. I could get run over. There's more chance of that. *The Guardian*

(Online Edition), http://www.guardian.co.uk/uk_news/story/0,3604, 984433,00.html (accessed July 16, 2003).

Centre for Genetics Education (2002). *Fact Sheet 36: Some Ethical Issues in Human Genetics*, http://www.genetics.com.au/Genetics2003/ Factsheets/36.asp (accessed July 7, 2003).

Codex Alimentarius Commission (2003a). *Guideline for the Conduct of Food Safety Assessment of Foods Produced Using Recombinant-DNA Microorganisms*, ftp://ftp.fao.org/es/esn/food/guide_mos_en.pdf (accessed August 18, 2009).

Codex Alimentarius Commission (2003b). *Principles for the Risk Analysis of Foods Derived from Modern Biotechnology*, ftp://ftp.fao.org/es/ esn/food/princ_gmfoods_en.pdf (accessed August 18, 2009).

Commission on Sustainable Development (2006). *Report of the Secretary-General: Overview of Progress towards Sustainable Development*, http://www.un.org/esa/sustdev/documents/docs_csd14.shtml (accessed October 9, 2007).

Convention on Biodiversity Secretariat (2009, 14 May). *Clearing House Mechanism: Introduction*, http://www.cbd.int/chm/intro (accessed June 10, 2009).

Dando, M., for the British Medical Association (1999). *Biotechnology, Weapons and Humanity*. Amsterdam: Harwood Academic Publishers.

Denny, C. (2001). WTO relaxes rule on drugs patents. *The Guardian (Online Edition)*, http://www.guardian.co.uk/business/story/0,3604, 592565,00.html (accessed June 4, 2003).

Dinham, B. (1993). *The Pesticide Hazard: A Global Health and Environmental Audit*. London: Zed Books.

Department of Energy (2009). *Human Genome Project Information: Gene Therapy*, http://www.ornl.gov/sci/techresources/Human_Genome/ medicine/genetherapy.shtml (accessed October 15, 2009).

UK Department of Health (2003). *Our Inheritance, Our Future: Realising the Potential of Genetics in the NHS*. Genetics white paper, http:// www.doh.gov.uk/genetics/whitepaper.html (accessed July 17, 2003).

Food and Agriculture Organization (n.d.). *Special Programme for Food Security*, http://www.fao.org/spfs/en/ (accessed October 9, 2007).

Food and Agriculture Organization (2003). *The Scourge of "Hidden Hunger": Global Dimensions of Micronutrient Deficiencies*, ftp://ftp.fao.org/docrep/fao/005/y8346my8346m01.pdf (accessed August 27, 2009).

Food and Agriculture Organization (2009). *Background Document "More People Than Ever Are Victims of Hunger,"* http://www.fao.org/fileadmin/user_upload/newsroom/docs/Press%20release%20june-en.pdf (accessed August 27, 2009).

Franco, C. (2009). Billions for biodefense: federal agency biodefense funding, FY2009-FY2010. *Biosecurity and Bioterrorism: Biodefense Strategy, Practice and Science*, 7(3), 291–309.

Goonatilake, S. (1999). *Merged Evolution: Long Term Implications of Biotechnology and Information Technology.* Amsterdam: Gordon & Breech.

Grand Challenges in Global Health Programme (n.d.). *Challenge 9: Create a Full Range of Optimal, Bioavailable Nutrients in a Single Staple Plant Species*, http://www.grandchallenges.org/ImproveNutrition/Challenges/NutrientRichPlants/Pages/default.aspx (accessed October 15, 2009).

Griffits, J. S., Whitacre, J. L., Stevens, D. E., and Araion, R. V. (2001). Bt toxin resistance from loss of a putative carbohydrate-modifying enzyme. *Science*, 293, 60–64.

Hindmarsh, R., Lawrence, G., and Norton, J. (eds.) (1998). *Altered Genes, Reconstructing Nature: The Debate.* St. Leonards, Australia: Allen & Unwin.

Hubbard, R., and Wald, E. (1993). *Exploding the Gene Myth.* Boston, MA: Beacon Press.

Human Genetics Commission (2001). *Debating the Ethical Future of Human Genetics: First Annual Report of the Human Genetics Commission*, http://www.hgc.gov.uk/business_publications_annualreport_first.pdf (accessed July 17, 2003).

International Chamber of Commerce (2002). *A Global Roadmap for Modern Biotechnology*, http://www.iccwbo.org/home/environment/roadmap/roadmap.asp (accessed January 30, 2003).

International Committee of the Red Cross (2002). *Biotechnology, Weapons and Humanity: FAQ and References*, http://www.icrc.org/Web/Eng/

siteeng0.nsf/html/1F00E7AC049A4758C1256C300054ADC7?Open Document&Style=Custo_Final.3&View=defaultBody2 (accessed February 20, 2004).

International Service for the Acquisition of Agri-biotech Applications (2009). *Brief 41: Global Status of Commercialized Biotech/GM Crops: 2009,* http://www.isaaa.org/resources/publications/briefs/41/default.asp (accessed October 15, 2010).

Kitcher, P. (1996). *The Lives to Come: The Genetic Revolution and Human Possibilities.* London: Allen Lane/Penguin.

Knight, W. (2002, 30 October). Zambia bans GM food aid. *New Scientist. com News Service,* http://www.newscientist.com/hottopics/gm/gm.jsp?id=ns99992990 (accessed June 3, 2003).

Madeley, J. (1996). *Yours for Food: Plant Genetic Resources and Food Security.* London: Christian Aid.

Marvier, M., McCreedy, C., Regetz, J., and Kareiva, P. (2007). A metaanalysis of effects of Bt cotton and maize on nontarget invertebrates. *Science,* **316,** 1475–1477.

McDowell, N. (2003, 15 January). New cancer case halts US gene therapy trials. *New Scientist.com News Service,* http://www.newscientist.com/news/news.jsp?id=ns99993271 (accessed June 2, 2003).

Meselson, M. (2000). Averting the hostile exploitation of biotechnology. *CBW Conventions Bulletin,* **48,** 16–19, http://www.fas.harvard.edu/~hsp/bulletin/cbwcb48.pdf (accessed June 3, 2003).

National Agricultural Statistics Service (n.d.). *Agricultural Chemical Use Database,* http://www.pestmanagement.info/nass/index.html (accessed October 15, 2009).

National Human Genome Research Institute (2009, 10 September). *International HapMap Project Overview,* http://www.genome.gov/10001688 (accessed October 15, 2009).

National Institute of Allergy and Infectious Diseases (2002). *Biodefense Research Agenda for CDC Category A Agents: Responding through Research,* http://www.niaid.nih.gov/biodefense/research/biotresearchagenda.pdf (accessed June 3, 2003).

Organisation for Economic Co-operation and Development (1998). *21st Century Technologies: Promises and Perils of a Dynamic Future.* Paris: Author.

Pilnick, A. (2002). *Genetics and Society: An Introduction*. Buckingham: Open University Press.

Pray, C. E., and Naseem, A. (2007). Supplying crop biotechnology to the poor: opportunities and constraints. *Journal of Development Studies Special Issue: Transgenics and the Poor; Biotechnology in Development Studies*, 43(1), 192–217.

Prentis, S. (1984). *Biotechnology: A New Industrial Revolution*. London: Orbis.

Qaim, M. (2000). *Potential Impacts of Crop Biotechnology in Developing Countries.*, Frankfurt: Peter Lang.

Quist, D., and Chapela, I. H. (2001). Transgenic DNA introgressed into traditional maize landraces in Oaxaca, Mexico. *Nature,* 414, 541–543, http://www.nature.com/cgi-taf/Dynapage.taf?file=/nature/journal/v414/n6863/full/414541a-fs.html (accessed June 2, 2003).

Rifkin, J. (1998). *The Biotech Century: The Coming Age of Genetic Commerce*. London: Victor Gollancz.

Rissler, J., and Mellon, M. (1996). *The Ecological Risks of Engineered Crops*. Cambridge, MA: MIT Press.

Thies, J. E., and Devare, M. H. (2007). An ecological assessment of transgenic crops. *Journal of Development Studies Special Issue: Transgenics and the Poor; Biotechnology in Development Studies*, 43(1), 97–129.

UNICEF (n.d.). *Water, Environment and Sanitation,* http://www.unicef.org/wes/index.html.

United Nations General Assembly (1948). *Universal Declaration of Human Rights,* http://www.un.org/Overview/rights.html (accessed July 17, 2003).

Union of Concerned Scientists (2004). *Technical Paper No.7: Genetically Engineered Crops and Pesticide Use in the United States; The First Nine Years,* http://www.ucsusa.org/assets/documents/food_and_agriculture/benbrook.pdf (accessed October 15, 2009).

Union of Concerned Scientists (2009). *Failure to Yield: Evaluating the Performance of Genetically Engineered Crops,* http://www.ucsusa.org/assets/documents/food_and_agriculture/failure-toyield.pdf (accessed October 15, 2009).

World Health Organisation (n.d.). *Micronutrient Deficiencies: Vitamin A Deficiency,* http://www.who.int/nutrition/topics/vad/en/index.html (accessed September 10, 2007).

World Health Organisation (2002). *Genomics and World Health: Report of the Advisory Committee on Health Research.* Geneva: Author. http://www3.who.int/health_topics/genetic_techniques/en/ (accessed 29 May 2003).

World Health Organisation (2008a). *World Malaria Report 2008,* http://whqlibdoc.who.int/publications/2008/978924156397_eng.pdf (accessed August 27, 2009).

World Health Organisation (2008b). *Worldwide Prevalence of Anaemia Report 1993–2005,* http://www.who.int/vmnis/anaemia/prevalence/en/ (accessed August 27, 2009).

World Health Organisation (2009). *Countries Move toward More Sustainable Ways to Roll Back Malaria,* http://www.who.int/mediacentre/news/releases/2009/malaria_ddt_20090506/en/index.html (accessed August 27, 2009).

World Trade Organization (2001, 20 November). *Doha Ministerial Declaration,* http://www.wto.org/english/thewto_e/minist_e/min01_e/mindecl_e.htm (accessed August 27, 2009).

Young, E. (2002, 2 October). Malaria's deadly secrets laid bare. *New Scientist.Com News Service,* http://www.newscientist.com/news/news.jsp?id=ns99992874 (accessed May 29, 2003).

Yoxen, E. (1986). *The Gene Business: Who Should Control Biotechnology?* London: Free Association Books.

Zilberman, D., Ameden, H., and Qaim, M. (2007). The impact of agricultural biotechnology on yields, risks and biodiversity in low income countries. *Journal of Development Studies Special Issue: Transgenics and the Poor; Biotechnology in Development Studies,* 43(1), 63–78.

Rōnin

Lena Nguyen *

G LENN HARKAWAY WAS SHOT in open court yesterday.
I suppose he knew the risks. When you're the district
attorney (DA), there's a whole slew of people who want to kill
you: the friends and families of people you've put away, crazies,
and even vigilantes sometimes. I was right there, sitting next to
Glenn, when it happened.

It wasn't someone sitting in the gallery, like you'd expect;
there are bulletproof windows in front of the pews to prevent
that. It was a court clerk, a little red-headed guy, all angles and
nervousness. He was sitting in front of me, his fingers jabbing
away at his holo-keyboard. He was recording our prosecution
of Rick White, the kingpin of a local drug racket. At some point
in the afternoon Glenn got up to make a motion, the clerk
twitched, and suddenly there was a sound like a clap of thunder,
punching through the air next to my ear. The hot smell of cordite
filled my nose and mouth, and my eyes clouded over with saline.
When I could see again, Glenn was lying on the ground next to
me, his legs jutting out from under the table in unnatural slants.
The clerk tried to drop the gun and run.

Why did he do it? We still don't know. The little bastard
hasn't given up anything from his holding cell in Belle Reve. My
best guess is that he was bribed, or threatened, or thought he
knew enough about the courthouse to make good on his escape

*Cornell University, Creative Writing program in English Language and Litera-
ture, 250 Goldwin Smith Hall, Cornell University Ithaca, NY 14853-3201, USA
lena.dg.nguyen@gmail.com

after he killed Glenn. What he didn't expect was for Glenn to stay conscious enough to lunge out from under the table and seize his ankles, tripping him up so that the bailiff could sprint over and pin him down.

That was Glenn's mistake, I think. If he had just stayed under the table, nobody in the gallery would have seen what they saw. He could have waited until the courtroom was empty or for the medics to come along and tidy him up, and we could have dealt with the whole thing quietly. But he just had to come out and grab the asshole who shot him. I guess I don't blame him.

Today the papers are buzzing with what happened, the articles bulging with angry words like a swarm of bees living inside the paper. I'm one of the last residents in the city to get my news in print. They don't wrap the papers in plastic anymore, so the rain has the columns of ink running down the page in dark rivers. I can pick out "DA a Sham: 7 Years and 153 Cases in Jeopardy." That's all I need to see.

Tara comes out of my bedroom, wearing one of my old college shirts, which falls down past her knees. She's a yawn on legs, her feet so soft and delicate they look like they'll melt into the kitchen floor. Her dark feathery hair is spiky with sleep, and so black that I imagine it'll smudge away, charcoal-like, if I reach out and touch it.

"Cereal?" I ask.

"Please." She angles a chair toward me and waits while I pour her some biogen raisin bran, which I bought during a recent and hazy midlife crisis.

"Bran?" she says, looking down at the sullen brown lumps. "You're 33, Jim, at least 20 years too young for this crap."

I grunt and go back to staring at my sodden newspaper. Tara glances over and remarks through a mouthful, "So they're already talking about Glenn."

"What did you expect?" I wad up the paper and throw the ball at the waste incinerator next to the counter. It bounces off the rim, but the bin's sensors do a brief scan, and it picks up the wad anyway. Tara says, "Are you going into the office today?"

"I guess I have to," I answer heavily. "The fallout there—everywhere—is going to be . . ."

"A shitstorm?"

"Yeah."

She looks at me. "Are you sure?"

I shrug. "I guess."

This is how it works. Tara isn't my wife or my girlfriend or anything. I'm in nervous love with her, but all she wants to be is a lover, minus the love. At most, she likes to trade for sex, giving out advice and decisiveness so I can have some forward motion in my life. I tell myself that it's a good trade-off, a win-win.

I lie to myself a lot.

I suit up for the day, checking myself in the mirror and trying to predict which features the public will pick apart during their 24-hour media slaughterhouse. Tara disappears into the bathroom. She's an artist and doesn't adhere to any kind of coherent working schedule, which, as a concept, makes me deeply anxious. She lives three floors up, so she'll wend between my apartment and her own like a stray cat—vanishing one week, twining back in the next. Zero commitment, she likes to say. No collars.

As I'm leaving, she pokes her head out of the bathroom and stares at me with her smoky eyes. I try to smile. We don't kiss each other goodbye.

~

The first time I met Glenn, I noticed right away the look of coolness he generated, the air of quiet finesse, like he was always alert and on guard but was too polite to fully show it. His clothes were dark in tone, devoid of logos and brands—a no-name look. At first glance, you wouldn't have thought that he was capable of being a public figure, let alone the DA of one of the largest biodome cities in the world.

But there was something more to him, something beyond the dark, laconic clothing. He wasn't charismatic, exactly, but people felt flattered by his regard. He'd look at them as if he was really listening, as if what they were talking about was worthy of his full attention—though he would never say so exactly. People wanted to be attached to him. He exuded potential, though potential for what, no one really knew.

At the time, I was nothing more than one of the many assistant attorneys in the office, weedy and neurotic, used to going unnoticed. It was a surprise when Glenn walked up to me during his first tour of the place. He looked into my face and shook my hand. He said, "Why do you look away?"

"I get nervous," I tried to joke. "Big new celeb in the office. Can I get your autograph?"

He'd smiled, very faintly, and said, "You're one of the good ones."

After that, I would have followed him anywhere, a little rock in the tail of his comet.

~

I take the bullet train to work. The televisions in the train compartment flash Glenn's face across the screens, and I try not to look at them. There's a dense knot in my stomach, and my hands are hot with sweat.

There's a mob boiling outside the office building. People are already outraged enough to stand on the curb, screaming, red faced, chanting the word "andy" and other words I can't make out. I even recognize some of them. They're relatives of the criminals that Glenn (and I) have locked up over our illustrious careers. My shoulders bunch up as I slog through the crowd, expecting a hot flash of pain in my back, the meaty thud of a phantom bullet, or an unseen knife. But no one recognizes me in the angry crush of people, and I manage to get to the door and have a security guard let me in.

All the assistant attorneys are upstairs, wandering around like the victims of a natural disaster. No one seems to be fielding the calls that are pouring into the place, the ringing of the phones coughing on and on.

I clear my throat. "Anyone going to get those?"

Everyone turns to me. "No point," says one of the assistant district attorneys (ADAs). It's Brad, a puffy, bull-necked guy who I always thought was more suited to bartending than practicing law. He's holding a box of Glenn's desk junk and glares at me, as if daring me to stop him. "Picking up some damn phones isn't going to help. What *will* help is—"

"Put Glenn's stuff down," I say tiredly.

"Why? He's not going to need it."

I don't say anything. Everyone in the office is looking at me; I have to steel myself so I don't fidget. Glenn was always the center of attention, the one who was in charge. I was like an extension of him, helpful but unnoticed—like a prehensile tail. Now I'm the monkey, and I hate it.

"Well?" prods Brad.

"Look," I say. "Just because Glenn's, you know, whatever, doesn't mean he doesn't want his stuff—"

This sends Brad into apoplexy. Office toys tumble out of his arms like the victims of a gunfight scrambling to get out of the way.

"*Glenn's a fucking robot,*" he explodes. "He doesn't need any goddamn paperweights! He doesn't need goddamn *anything*—"

"There's no need for that kind of language," someone cuts in.

And there's Glenn, standing in the doorway behind me. I almost don't recognize him at first. His face is the same—the aristocratic nose, the straight dark hair—but something about him seems deflated, his body even thinner than usual. There's a lump under his suit at chest level, where they hastily patched up the bullet hole with synthetic wadding. One of his top buttons is undone, and there's the telltale metallic gleam of alloy under his shirt.

After a pause, he walks further into the room. No one speaks. We're all looking for the signs, the signs that everyone uses to pick out androids, like the ones that operate as sex workers or prison guards. Those androids, the regular ones, all have this strange, lightly bobbing way of moving, as if the internal rotors aren't moving fast enough—and there's a slow drag of the eyes.

Glenn shows none of this. He walks just like a normal person, and if it weren't for the metal showing, I'd forget again that he isn't.

He notices all of us looking at the unbuttoned part of his shirt, but doesn't move to cover it up. Instead, he says, "I'm deeply sorry, everyone. The deception was never meant to go this far."

Still no one speaks. Everyone is gawping at him, not sure how to reconcile the image of the serious man who's been our boss for seven years with the idea that he's a machine. There's a cottony, uncomfortable silence, pressing everyone down into the carpet, before Glenn takes a few slow steps to the nearest chair and makes a crumpling movement into it.

Then he says, "I mean it. It really wasn't my intention."

"Whose intention was it, then?" I ask, my voice like a teenager's, a high, incredulous squawk.

Glenn looks at me, his green eyes—Glass? Plastic? Liquid somehow?—clear and perspicacious. He doesn't answer. Brad butts in, "So what happens now?"

Glenn's eyes turn to him. "I resign, obviously. Or was that not what you were referring to?"

Brad looks angry, livid even, but seven years of being in awe of Glenn is hard to shake. "I mean the people who were convicted. By you. They'll want to give them retrials. Most of them will probably walk."

Glenn says, "We'll think on that." He stares straight at Brad for a moment, unmoving, and for an unnerving second I wonder if he's shut down. Then he blinks, and I ask myself, *Does he do it out of habit, or do they program blinking into him?*

Then: *Stop it. Stop. Once you start down that road, you never get off.*

"Jim," Glenn says, "may I speak to you in private?"

Swallow. "Sure," I manage. My throat is dry and sticky at the same time. I feel feverish, as if I've been cut all over with glass and inflamed. We go into Glenn's office, which has already been ransacked by Brad, and sit down in his sleek leather chairs. I feel myself go cold when he chooses the guest chair, leaving me the one behind the desk. His chair. The DA's chair.

"I'm sure you have a lot of questions," he says after a long pause that leaves me looking at everything but him. He sighs at me. "Jim. I am truly sorry."

"Okay."

"Do you want to ask me anything?"

I'm numb, vinegary with shock and maybe hatred. I answer cautiously, "I don't know yet."

He nods. "Alright. Then I'll give you the bare bones of it. How does that sound?" He doesn't wait for me to reply. "Several years ago, a certain research institute—and I won't say which—wondered if it was possible to create an android who could understand complex human values. Up until then, androids were only capable of delivery work, sanitation jobs, jobs that—" He hesitates. "Jobs that *humans* didn't want. But the technology was available, the technology to create and explore synthetic intelligence."

"So they made you."

"So the story goes." He looks thoughtful for a moment, and there's the briefest instinct, the quickest twitch of residual memory that almost makes me ask him if he wants to bail on work, get some sim-coffee, or go to the tennis club. Then he says, "So they made me. Then they placed me in a law firm that had already given consent, to see how I would interact in that environment. To see if someone like me could process human laws and ethics and moral quandaries."

"And?"

He smiles thinly. "Well, I was elected DA."

"You're very full of yourself."

He shrugs. "I was only meant to assume the role of a regular lawyer. No one expected . . . Well, it was never anyone's intention."

"You keep saying that," I say, annoyed, but he gives me such a bland look that I know picking a fight with him won't lead anywhere. I straighten in the chair and yank on the end of my tie. "So. So where's this institute of yours now? Is it going to own up?"

He waves his hand. "It dissolved years ago. I've been on my own for quite some time—since I was elected, in fact. They didn't want to risk anyone claiming that I was being used for political gain. And even if they hadn't disbanded, they didn't do anything illegal. There are no laws against androids running for office."

This is ridiculous, I think. *There are no laws because there are no androids that are capable of running for office.*

Except you.

But this would just feed his ego, if he even has one, so I say nothing. Glenn continues, "Enough with the past. We need to talk about the future."

"What *about* the future?" I ask him incredulously. "Aren't you going to turn yourself in? For police protection, at least?

The whole city's in a frenzy. They want your blood—or oil, or whatever."

"Don't worry about that. Focus on what you're going to do about the convicted."

"What *I'm* going to do!"

He turns the corners of his mouth down, and again he is simply Glenn, *human* Glenn, the Glenn of my memories: straightforward, no-nonsense, kind-of-funny-in-a-flat-way Glenn. I feel sweat forming in patches against the back of my shirt. Here's a guy that I've invited to my apartment on Sunday afternoons, had drinks with, played holo-chess against. What did all of that mean to him? What does anything mean now?

"You're acting DA now," Glenn tells me, in his low, crisp voice. "That means you have a responsibility to see things through. Whatever I am, whatever problems others may now have with me, you can't deny that every single person we've brought to justice deserved to be convicted. Vincent Mazurek. John Fulbreech. Lucia Lockheed. We—all of us—worked for months to prove that they were people who deserved to be sentenced. *Needed* to be, for the good of others. My nature doesn't change that."

I can't answer. My hands are open, turned upward, helplessly signaling, *I don't know what in hell you want me to do.* I don't want to respond to him. I recognize Glenn-magic when I see it, after years of watching him perform in court; I know his tricks. If I give him a response, he'll go after it like a dog with a bone, worrying away at my feeble confidence until I'm convinced that up is down and the New Packers are going to win the playoffs.

"You can't let all of our work go to waste," Glenn presses.

"Didn't you already do that for us?" I ask.

He looks down and starts picking invisible lint off his sleeve, something he does when he's thinking. I have to ask myself again if he was programmed to do it.

He drops a stray thread in the trashcan. "Has the mayor said anything?"

How should I know? "I just got here," I answer irritably. His artificial gaze swings up, landing on the side of my face like a searchlight. I hesitate, then relent, "He called last night. To say that we should hold off on a press conference. He didn't say anything else." Outside, the phones are still going off like war sirens.

Glenn's mouth twists. "They're going to use you as a scapegoat, Jim. You're second-in-command—they can easily divorce themselves of the situation and throw you to the wolves."

"It's not that bad."

"No? The public is very angry."

I look down at the corner of his desk. There's a crumpled wrapper underneath it. It must be Brad's; Glenn is—was—too much of a neat-freak to allow that kind of thing in his own work space.

"I think you should leave," I say to my shoes.

He nods, standing, but doesn't make a move toward the door. The lump in his chest is more prominent than ever. He leans over the desk, his long, pale hand flattened against it, and I look down at his skin and see real pores. "Are you sure you don't have any questions, Jim?"

He waits, but I can't bring myself to say anything. I have many questions, innumerable questions, but they're all stuffed up inside of me, smashed together like wet tissues balled into a pulp. *Is this a joke?* I want to ask, but I know it's not. I was in the courtroom. I saw what he really was.

"Jim? No questions?"

I think, *Here's a question for you, jackass. How could you have been an android all along? How did I never notice? How could you have been my boss, my friend?*

How could you do this to me?

Glenn is turning away. He opens the door to his office, and all of the ADAs flinch away from him. We watch as he makes his way back to the lobby door, stiffly, like a bona fide combat veteran, and I find myself straining to catch any mechanical sounds coming from him: gears grinding, boxes overheating. But there is nothing, and he says nothing. The door shuts with a smooth little click.

Brad turns to me. "Did you know, Jim?" he demands. "Did you know all along?"

"No," I tell him tiredly. "No, I never knew." But it's hard to say it. As with all knowledge, once you know something, you can't imagine how it was before you knew. It reaches backward; you can't remember what things were like before. Like stage magic, knowledge of something takes place before your very eyes, but you never see it coming. You were looking elsewhere.

～

The day that Glenn promoted me to his second-in-command, six months after taking office, I was so stunned that I didn't speak for well over an hour. Everyone else in the office was appalled; guys like me never got promoted to executive ADA. The ones who got promoted were charismatic, aggressive—essentially, the antithesis of whatever I was. I still thought it was a sad prank until Glenn pulled me aside at the end of the day.

"What's the matter?" he asked.

I shrugged. "Just surprised, is all."

Glenn smiled, very cool and unconcerned, and said, "You're smart, and you care about people. I have faith in you."

"I think that's the first time anyone's ever said that to me," I admitted.

"Well, get used to it," he answered, heading toward the elevator. "From now on, I'm counting on you to have my back."

And from that day on, I did. Now, looking back, I wonder what it was that made him choose me. Was it a calculated risk, an analysis that saw something more than the human eye could catch? Or was it the result of a faulty algorithm, a stray defect in the programming—a decision made by a machine that should only handle hauling garbage and doing math?

~

"You're going to have to take a side eventually," Tara tells me when I call her. It's time to leave work, and the mob outside has been joined by a horde of reporters. I can see them through the office windows, lined up like a firing squad. I'm panicking because I'm looking at my notes, and they're just blank sheets of paper. No one in the office is trying to help me. A lot of them have taken off to go drink at a bar, and I didn't stop them when they left. None of my superiors have said a word either; they've gone dark, radio silence.

"I thought politicians aren't supposed to take sides," I say, cramming a piece of mango into my mouth. Every time I get a craving for an e-cig, I just eat mangoes.

"You're not a politician, you're a lawyer, and lawyers always take sides." Her voice is patient, but I can tell she's annoyed; I probably interrupted her during some meditative inspiration-seeking, or hunting-for-dead-animals something. (That's her latest art project. Painting has been dead for years, so Tara finds animal carcasses and drives them out to the desert and arranges them into giant words. She does this so that when the flies and buzzards come, she can take a bird's-eye snapshot from a helicopter and show the world some really ugly, living sentences. Recently she put one up on my fridge, a grisly portrait of the word LOVE, and said, "To remind you that love is dead, Jim.")

"Maybe I can just say I'm sick."

"Man up, James."

We end the call on that note. *Man up.*

Man up, I tell myself as I ease out the door. There are lights shining on me in waves of heat, driving me back into catastrophic memories of playing Mr. Bingley in the ninth-grade production of *Pride and Prejudice.* Sweat starts to pour down me in sheets. I keep thinking about the after-show party where I ate Stacey Price's lacy butter cookies and she kissed me while the cookies were still in my mouth; I passed out from delayed nerves.

The first question whizzes past me and punches into the wall. "Did you know that Glenn Harkaway was an android?"

"No," I say very faintly, despite myself. I clear my throat and repeat at the same airless volume, "No. Nobody in the office knew."

"Did the mayor know? What about anyone involved in his campaign for DA seven years ago?"

I don't know this one. "No comment."

"Where is the robot now?"

My brain is working furiously, but it's like a jackhammer pounding away at something that will never yield. I start fast-walking. "No comment."

"As the executive ADA, what are your thoughts on the men you've helped Harkaway send to prison? Are their sentences still valid, since they weren't even prosecuted by a human being?"

"Will they be retried?"

"Do you believe that a machine could really understand the nuances of justice and human morality? Enough to fairly indict real people?"

"Is there anyone else in your office or the local government who is also an android?"

I'm running now, and shoving, hot-eyed and blind with panic. *No comment,* I chant, over and over in a mantra. That's my whole life now. *No comment. No comment. No comment.*

~

Eventually I'm able to get away and scuttle to Cuppajoe, the café where Glenn and I used to go once a week to drink coffee and toke up. He did eat, Glenn, and drink and smoke—very politely, as if he were always standing on ceremony. I wonder now how he did it. No other android that I know of can eat or smoke. It's no wonder he never seemed stoned. I always just thought he had a high tolerance.

As I let the sim-coffee work its way through my veins, I lie back into one of the egg-shaped chairs and think about Glenn. How would he have handled the press, before everyone found out he was an android? What would he have said if he were under fire?

"You think too much of what other people think of you," he said to me once. I was sulking over a blunder I'd made during one of his public statements. "In the end, all that matters is what you think of yourself and if you can be proud of your actions and what you've done. People forget. Life goes on."

"I don't know how you can be so casual about all of this," I'd groaned.

He gave me one of his half-smiles and passed over the blunt. "I have to be," he'd answered. "It's one of those tricks you learn in the trade. You'll get used to it."

Thanks a lot, Glenn.

I drag a hand down my face, pulling at the bags under my eyes. I never should have gotten the position. Glenn had told me he had needed a right-hand man, not someone who would always be gunning for his job, and for a long time I'd taken it as a compliment.

But what do you do when you're the right hand of a machine? What do you do when you get cut off and everyone wants to pretend that you're as good as the missing body? And worse, what do you do if you *know* you can't be as good as the body, which is nothing more than a nest of wires and glowing lights?

Outside of Cuppajoe, there's a ring of people standing around a delivery droid. It's built to look like a slender blonde woman, but you can tell right away that it's a bot: its movements are jerky and unsure, and it has that blank unseeing stare that the older models have. Its bag of packages is spilling at its feet.

I hear someone say as I pass, "You think you're better than real people, too?"

The android's eyes are lowered in a display of deference. "I don't think at all," it answers humbly.

The mass of people fall on it like a ton of bricks. A lot of them are teenagers, angry youths who are just looking for an excuse for destruction. But the robot gets torn to pieces, synthetic skin fluttering in scraps, metal skull being bashed against the wall. It doesn't resist. It's not allowed to. I stand and watch until some city patrolmen come by and chase the attackers off for destruction of property.

A pile of hair and metal is all that's left in their wake, along with the trampled bag of packages. As I look on, the android's glass eyes swivel wildly from within its ruined face and seem to skewer me. *Why didn't you help me, Jim?* they accuse. *Where's your humanity?*

~

Glenn was the one who introduced me to Tara. She told me later that she'd lost interest straightaway, that she'd thought I was a "dweeb." Our first date was a disaster. I was so nervous around her—fiercely beautiful, contemptuous, casually defiant—that I never even got to tell her that I was the executive ADA (my sole winning point). Even when we'd found that we lived in the same building, she hadn't seemed interested.

I went moping to Glenn about it the day afterward. He didn't know her well—they were acquaintances through some series of fundraisers and auctions at the art gallery—but he knew what the problem was immediately.

"I'm too boring for someone like her," I said. "Give me someone, you know, *plainer.*"

"Go back to her," Glenn said, exactly as if he were advising me to go to the doctor, "and speak your mind. Tell her exactly what it is you're thinking. She's not the type who enjoys posturing or niceties. You'll win her over by being forthright."

He fed me glasses of Glenfiddich whiskey, patiently, until I worked up my nerve. Before I left, I gave him a sloppy hug and said, "You're my best friend."

Glenn smiled faintly and said, "I know."

I don't remember what I said to Tara. It must have been something that impressed her enough to let me in, and it must have been devoid of enough commitment for her to feel secure enough to let me stay. For weeks after, I tortured myself over what the magic words were, even as Tara continued to open her door for me. I asked Glenn over and over what I said, marveling and despairing all at once. His only response was to shrug a little and say, "The words are there, Jim. You just need the courage to let them out."

~

The fallout from Glenn's scandal causes society to erupt like a summer bonfire. A rash of paranoia breaks out, with everyone wondering who *else* could be a robot, and the Humanists slinging hysteria at every turn. My higher-ups, mainly the attorney general and the mayor, continue to hold off on a press conference. They also ignore my calls. Like Glenn predicted, they take pains to stay in the shadows, throwing me further into the spotlight— and the only thing I can do is dance around inevitable disaster.

No one knows whom to point fingers at. The group who built Glenn really has dissolved, allowing him to go out into the world to be his own man. Like Adam being cast out of the Garden, Glenn was turned loose, allowed to go rogue: masterless, his actions as DA were entirely his own, and he seems to be the only one accountable. But he has disappeared, and no one knows if the police should be searching for him because they don't know if what he did is a crime.

The families of the convicted want justice—and blood. They're screaming for the release of their loved ones, who were locked away by a cold, heartless machine who didn't know any better. They neglect to mention that their beloved criminals were put in jail for being proved, beyond a shadow of a doubt—*my* doubt, anyway—to be guilty of crimes like serial rape and child homicide.

"Would you want a computer deciding whether your son would die in prison?" a protester blares at me when I walk to Cuppajoe. "What about a geniusphone, or the program that chooses the lottery numbers? This is crazy! This needs to be fixed!"

But by whom? I want to ask him. Whose heads do you want to roll? No one knows, and it's like throwing a bucket of blood into the water. With nothing real to feed on, the sharks start tearing themselves apart.

This undirected backlash causes massive dropouts at the office. Brad is one of the first to go. When he hands me his letter of resignation, having printed it out on our creamiest stock paper instead of just e-mailing it, he gives me one last parting shot:

"How's it feel, playing second fiddle to a bot this whole time?"

I want to say something scathing, like the fact that he was even lower than me in relation to Glenn, so he was playing something like *sixth* fiddle to a bot. But he leaves to collect his things before I can say it, and then the sting sets in. I have always been considered inferior to Glenn, but for me it was just status quo. I could never resent him for it. Glenn was that friend who always got As without even going to class, while you studied your ass off and only managed to scrape a B. It was just the way of things. I had always told myself that it wasn't my fault, or his. That some people were just born certain ways, and there was nothing either of us could do about it.

Now I don't know if it's insulting, his being a machine, or if it just makes sense. I feel the knot in my stomach tighten.

That night, Tara finds out about the dropouts and calls them a bunch of blood-sucking bastards. I agree morosely, and seeing my preoccupation, she slides under the sheets and distracts me with her mouth until I want to shout. Then she comes back up and says, "My show at the gallery is opening next week."

"Oh," I say, light-headed. "Are you asking me to come?"

She gives me a look, very cat-like and quietly scathing, and I sink back onto the pillows. There are some very firm boundaries between Tara and myself; for instance, she has never allowed me to come to her art shows, because it would be too "intimate." I never argue with this because I get the feeling that, at the first sign of real attachment, she'll pelt out the door like someone fleeing the scene of a crime.

I dared to ask her once why she acted like this—what she was so afraid of. She'd said that where she'd grown up, outside of the biodome, everything was a trade. People had to survive on their ability to trade. For information, for supplies, for favors, for attention. Love was useless because it led you into dumb trades. Love made you give too much away.

"I'd give it back, though," I'd said. "I'd make it fair."

She'd laughed. "Oh, Jim," she'd said. "You don't know what you're talking about."

Then she'd said I wasn't allowed to come to her galleries.

Out of habit, I think about talking to Glenn about this. Then I feel a tide of redness surge up within me. My face goes acidic, and I realize that, for the first time in my life, I am feeling true hatred.

I have to hire a temporary security guard to accompany me home every day after work. There is an enormous upsurge of attacks on robots, and soon the streets are littered with broken pieces of metal and hardware. The same question is hammered through the city: how could a robot ever judge human beings? How could a machine presume to understand human emotions and thoughts and ideas?

Sometimes I agree with this. But then I think about Glenn sitting quietly on the couch, holding a beer and listening while I talked to him about Tara and TV shows and how much I miss books in print. "Me too," he would say feelingly. Then I don't know what to think, and I hate him a little more.

One night, before I leave the office, I get a call on my wrist phone from an unknown number. I pick up without thinking about it, only belatedly realizing that it could be a death threat. But the voice on the other line is familiar.

"Good evening, Jim."

Everything outside my office door goes quiet; there's a rush of static in my ears. Heat swamps on my face. I manage to croak, stupidly, "Hey, Glenn."

"How are things going?"

I'm sitting at my desk, in the middle of packing my things up for the day. Without realizing it, I start to knead the paper I'm holding into a damp ball, the lump in my stomach thickening. "Pretty shitty, if I'm going to be perfectly honest."

He sighs. "I thought so."

"Where are you?"

"Someplace hidden," he answers, with typical succinctness. "I called because I'm worried."

"About me?" I try for sarcasm. "Gee, thanks."

"Not your well-being, exactly." I'm straining again for some hint that his voice isn't a human's voice, that it's sound manipulated by speakers or boxes or whatever it is, but his tone is perfectly clear. "You can take care of yourself, Jim," he continues. "I'm more concerned about your lack of response over the convicted. You need to get out there and make a statement."

Wow. "I'm not allowed to hold a press conference yet."

"According to whom?"

"The *mayor*, Glenn." My collar feels too tight. "You're not DA anymore. Why don't you give it a rest?"

There's a rustling sound, and I hear him exhale through his nose. I can tell he's reconsidering his plan of action. "Look," he says, "I'm sorry. I was just hoping we could talk. I realize that you're angry and that you must have more questions. I want to do you the courtesy of answering them."

A laugh bubbles up in my throat, low and bitter. "You're an asshole, Glenn. Stop trying to play the nice guy." He doesn't say anything. I steamroll on: "You're a goddamn asshole. How do you think it makes me feel, finding out that my best friend has been a machine all these years? How pathetic do you think I feel? It's like everything that you influenced in my life, everything you helped me out with, everything you were responsible for— all of that might as well have been me talking to an imaginary friend. None of it means anything."

"Jim, I understand you're conflicted—"

"The whole time you were just lying. Playing along. It's inhuman, Glenn."

"Listen," Glenn says, his voice growing clipped in the way it does when he's irritated. "I just want to make sure—"

"Make sure of what?" I demand. "Make sure I do the right thing? If you're so unsure, why'd you put this all on me in the first place?"

He doesn't say anything. I feel as if my bones have been lined with gunpowder and Glenn's lit the fuse. My blood fizzes.

"Why'd you even pick me, Glenn?" I ask, my voice sandy and mean. "Why was I the one who had to take your place? Why am I the one who inherits your shit? Why me?"

"I chose you," Glenn says calmly, "because you were the right man for the job."

I hang up. Before I leave, I toss my wrist phone into a drawer in my desk and lock it away.

That night, a news story breaks on the TVs in the bullet train. At first there's so much noise and shouting coming from the screens that I can't make out what the reporter is saying. The camera zooms in on unrecognizable metal wreckage: long pieces of alloy, straggling wires like clutches of black worms.

"Another robot killing," says my bodyguard, looking up at the screen.

"Yeah." I only feel tired and miserable, hyperdistant from what's going on around me. I watch as a crowd of people stomps on the remains, grinding the whole mess into smaller metal shards. "Jesus, they really tore it apart."

The news feed on his wrist phone lights up, and he checks it briefly. Then he says, "You don't have your phone on you?"

"No. What happened?"

He thrusts the little display at me. *Robot Glenn Harkaway destroyed,* it reads. More words flash past: *The android, former district attorney, was spotted walking west through Lincoln Park and was attacked by a group of angry civilians. By the time police arrived on scene, the android was totally beyond repair.*

On TV, splinters of what used to be Glenn glow like stars in the orange flush of the street lights.

I feel cold dread. Lincoln Park is the park next to my apartment.

I go home not really thinking about anything. It's the night of Tara's art show opening. She comes into the apartment to find me sitting at the counter, staring at the mug that used to be Glenn's. He always washed that mug himself because he saw how I wash all of my other cups; he used to say he'd die of plague if he kept using my dishes.

"Oh, honey," Tara says when she sees me staring at the chips on the rim of the mug. She puts her arms around me and runs her cheek against my hair. "Oh, sweetie. It's sad, isn't it?"

"I guess," I say, and for a moment I let her warmth soak into me, the feel of her spongy and sweet and comfortable. Then I get a whiff of something under the scent of her hair, something musky and dark. Men's cologne. A man's scent.

I push her off without saying anything. She just looks at me with her large, smudgy eyes, her mouth making a little pink frown. I say, my voice fricative, "Don't."

"Don't?"

"Don't."

I close my eyes. My hand curls hard around the mug. I'm suddenly gloriously angry, furious even, furious with Glenn for dying, furious with him for being a robot. Furious with Tara for being more of a robot than he was.

"Don't act like you care if you don't," I rasp.

Tara's mouth is pulling lower and lower. "What are you saying?"

"You don't care about Glenn," I say, my breath coming rough and shallow. "No one does."

"But I care about *you*, Jim."

The blood is pumping through me, bright and fast. I want to tell her that I hate that she goes with other men, hate that she won't let me come close, hate that she thinks love is dead. I want to tell her I won't go along with it. I want to tell her that she can't say that she cares—that no one in the world cares except me.

Instead I blurt out, "You're just like a robot. You go through the motions, but you don't feel anything. What's wrong with you?"

She doesn't say anything. My voice rises like an overflowing river cresting a dam: "Why can't you feel? Why can I? Why can't you love me the way I love you?"

And there it is: stupidity in its finest form. When I say it, I have the vague and fuzzy notion that my newfound aggression will seduce Tara into staying with me forever. I nearly even say that I want to marry her. But she's gone before I do. The door rattles shut behind her.

I turn back to the mug with a sense of disappointment and faint relief. In the darkness of the apartment, all I can see are the soggy, moldering newspapers piling up on my kitchen table. It's been raining a lot lately.

~

In the morning, I call a press conference. I tell the reporters that I'll come and talk to them at Lincoln Park at ten. I don't bother going in to work.

Then I go and sit at the foot of the statue where I said I'd be. The statue is a depiction of Protagoras, which makes a hollow laugh simmer low in my stomach. I do have to smile. Press conferences usually come with stages, lecterns, and prepared speeches. I sit on the base of a statue streaked with bird shit, dressed in a button-down and some slacks. I haven't showered or shaved. My hands are empty.

There is a trail of fine powder made of crushed glass that arcs around the statue. I wonder if any of it was once a part of Glenn's body. I pick up a sliver of metal lying next to my shoe and hold it to the light.

A fuzz of shadow has covered my thoughts, but it can't subdue my questions. What was the thing that drove Glenn through the years? If he was really free to do what he wanted, if no one was telling him what to do, or programming commands into his head—what was it that made him tick?

When the reporters arrive, I drop the piece of metal and pin it beneath my foot. The air goes quiet and still, even though the journalists are pressing toward me, clamoring with questions, fighting each other like dogs over scraps of meat. Their collective attention is like a small white sun gathering at the center of my body. I steel myself.

"I'm only going to say three things today," I say. My voice, usually thin and reedy, has taken on a strange timbre. The journalists quiet.

"First thing," I say, gathering steam. "Glenn Harkaway. He wasn't a man in the true sense of the word, but he was more of a man than a lot of people I know. Including myself." I falter when a ripple goes through the little crowd but force myself to continue. "Glenn fought for what was right. I know now that he was a machine, but he was capable of knowing right and wrong, and he always chose, of his own free will, to do what was right. He was a great person and a good friend."

My face is shining with sweat, but I'm afraid to wipe it. The journalists are so transfixed that they're staring at me as if I'm a lab rat, as if they're scientists who are fascinated by what I'm going to do next.

"Second thing," I say. "And I'm speaking as the acting DA in Glenn's place. Even if Glenn was an android, that doesn't affect the cases of the men whom we've convicted in the past. It was the judge and jury of each case—who were all humans—who decided those men's guilt and condemned them. Glenn just put forth arguments and used very real legal knowledge. He did what all robots are supposed to do, which is to apply the skills they're programmed with. He was given a job, and he did it. His ability to convince the court only shows how exceptional he was.

But it was humans who decided that he was right, and decided to send those people to prison. So Glenn's nature has nothing to do with the actual convictions. It would make no sense for those people to be retried."

Immediately, I'm bombarded with a volley of questions and demands, most of them asking me to clarify what I've just said. Some people in the crowd who aren't journalists start hurling insults at me, and threats. They start screaming my name. But I don't leave. My back is straight.

"Third thing," I say. "Glenn gave his life continuing to do what he believed in. He died for what he thought was right. He didn't have to, but he chose to put himself at risk because he believed in things bigger than himself: justice, fairness, and the law. And I'll continue his fight if I have to."

The crowd surges. The bystanders who have been howling my name break through the line of journalists, jabbing fingers at me, spittle flying from their mouths. They shove their faces into mine, and I don't move. In a matter of seconds, some policemen—the same ones, I want to believe, that chased off Glenn's attackers—snag me by the collar and start dragging me backward.

"Fourth thing," I shout at one of the cameras. "Tara, I love you, and I'm not sorry for it."

I let the police bear me through the lake of human bodies. A few fists catch me around the shoulders and head, but I don't care. I feel strangely weightless, my vision hyperclear and surreally sharp. My body is thrumming like a plucked string. I'm grinning. The sun lances through the clouds and falls on my face like a warm hand.

Glenn was right, I think, feeling something loosen within me: a hidden key turning in its lock. Glenn was right all along. The words were there. I just needed to let them out.

～

The mayor, of course, has me fired immediately. He actually wants me to be visited by a psychiatrist to validate claims that I'm mentally unhinged: it's the only way to explain my unthinkable comments to the press. A machine, being a great person and a good friend? An android having any concept of morality and fighting for justice? They're the ideas of a lunatic.

I more or less expected this reaction. Sometimes I'm not entirely sure that I am sane, that I haven't simply snapped under the pressure. I'm concerned by my own lack of concern over losing my job. But I try to bear it up with grace—the kind that Glenn would have shown in my position.

Before I leave the office forever, the remaining ADAs let me know that they've pitched in money to buy Glenn a grave. It's an unmarked stone in a cemetery outside the city. What we could have buried there was sucked up by a street sweeper and trashed in the city dump. But in their own small way, they're telling me that they agree with what I said.

I discover Tara a few weeks after I leave the office. I open my door to find her standing in the hallway, eyes dangling. She's not wearing makeup. She looks limp and worn out. I step back to let her in.

Once inside, she falls back against the door and her downcast eyes flicker up to mine.

"I saw what you said," she says thickly. "On TV."

"So did everybody else in the country," I answer. I try to smile.

Tara bows her head. The light from the kitchen falls against the door and seems to stab her, and words flow out of her like blood: "Can I stay?"

When I nod, she goes to the fridge and rips up her picture of the carcasses.

That night I dream about Glenn and the day he was shot in the courtroom. Beneath my closed eyes I see myself ducking under the table to see if he's okay. I see him lying on the floor with his eyes open, the hole in his chest smoking, the wound splayed out in a blast radius. Coolant is leaking out of him in clear puddles. His metal ribs have punched out through his skin. I can see a small, whirring ball of light in the ruin of his chest, spinning and pulsing through him, and Glenn is smiling because the bullet has missed his heart.

Appendix

76 Reasonable Questions to Ask about Any Technology (by Jacques Ellul)

Ecological

1. What are its effects on the health of the planet and of the person?
2. Does it preserve or destroy biodiversity?
3. Does it preserve or reduce ecosystem integrity?
4. What are its effects on land?
5. What are its effects on wildlife?
6. How much and what kind of waste does it generate?
7. Does it incorporate the principles of ecological design?
8. Does it break the bond of renewal between humans and nature?
9. Does it preserve or reduce cultural diversity?
10. What is the totality of its effects, its "ecology"?

Social

11. Does it serve community?
12. Does it empower community members?
13. How does it affect our perception of our needs?
14. Is it consistent with the creation of a communal, human economy?
15. What are its effects on relationships?
16. Does it undermine conviviality?
17. Does it undermine traditional forms of community?

18. How does it affect our way of seeing and experiencing the world?
19. Does it foster a diversity of forms of knowledge?
20. Does it build on, or contribute to, the renewal of traditional forms of knowledge?
21. Does it serve to commodify knowledge or relationships?
22. To what extent does it redefine reality?
23. Does it erase a sense of time and history?
24. What is its potential to become addictive?

Practical

25. What does it make?
26. Who does it benefit?
27. What is its purpose?
28. Where was it produced?
29. Where is it used?
30. Where must it go when it's broken or obsolete?
31. How expensive is it?
32. Can it be repaired? By an ordinary person?

Moral

33. What values does its use foster?
34. What is gained by its use?
35. What are its effects beyond its utility to the individual?
36. What is lost in using it?
37. What are its effects on the least advantaged in society?

Ethical

38. How complicated is it?
39. What does it allow us to ignore?
40. To what extent does it distance agent from effect?
41. Can we assume personal or communal responsibility for its effects?

42. Can its effects be directly apprehended?
43. What ancillary technologies does it require?
44. What behavior might it make possible in the future?
45. What other technologies might it make possible?
46. Does it alter our sense of time and relationships in ways conducive to nihilism?

Vocational

47. What is its impact on craft?
48. Does it reduce, deaden, or enhance human creativity?
49. Is it the least imposing technology available for the task?
50. Does it replace or does it aid human hands and human beings?
51. Can it be responsive to organic circumstances?
52. Does it depress or enhance the quality of goods?
53. Does it depress or enhance the meaning of work?

Metaphysical

54. What aspect of the inner self does it reflect?
55. Does it express love?
56. Does it express rage?
57. What aspect of our past does it reflect?
58. Does it reflect cyclical or linear thinking?

Political

59. Does it concentrate or equalize power?
60. Does it require or institute a knowledge elite?
61. Is it totalitarian?
62. Does it require a bureaucracy for its perpetuation?
63. What legal empowerments does it require?
64. Does it undermine traditional moral authority?
65. Does it require military defense?
66. Does it enhance or serve military purposes?

67. How does it affect warfare?
68. Is it massifying?
69. Is it consistent with the creation of a global economy?
70. Does it empower transnational corporations?
71. What kind of capital does it require?

Aesthetic

72. Is it ugly?
73. Does it cause ugliness?
74. What noise does it make?
75. What pace does it set?
76. How does it affect the quality of life (as distinct from the standard of living)?

Index

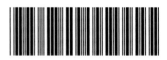